AERYON

WELLNESS

navigating perimenopause

This book is dedicated to my daughter and to all young women, so that with information like this and open conversations, they may feel supported and less alone when navigating the pivotal journey of perimenopause.

Welcome

Here's to a Beautiful New Beginning

Welcome to "Navigating Perimenopause," your guide to stepping into the second half of your glorious life. This transition can be daunting and filled with unknowns, but it also can be an exciting new chapter. As you journey through midlife, remember that it's not an end but rather a beautiful beginning.

I get it. More than 15 years ago, I had a health crisis. I was exhausted, my anxiety was through the roof, my periods were heavy and inconsistent, my sleep was sporadic, my skin was dry (ALL OVER!), my libido was non-existent and my lab work indicated I was starting early perimenopause. More importantly, I did not feel like myself anymore.

Witnessing my mother's struggles with menopause, I realized that my condition was potentially on an even more difficult path, particularly concerning my post menopausal health. Motivated by this, I embarked on a journey to redefine my approach to nutrition, daily movement, stress management and sleep habits.

This also catalyzed me being an advocate for my health and wellness alongside a team of practitioners. However, as I looked on the market for a natural solution for additional support, I found nothing with clinical, validated doses made by women, to support my journey. This is when Aeryon Wellness Support Supplements was born.

Over the past several years, I have had the great pleasure of traveling across Canada speaking on women's health, connecting to women who are all feeling the same and looking for answers.

If my story resonates with you, you are in the right place. Aeryon Wellness is committed to supporting and empowering you in your health journey, especially during this transformative phase. This manual is designed to educate and equip you with practical action steps that will help you navigate perimenopause with grace and confidence. You're not alone in this journey; I will be here to lend a hand, guiding you toward feeling your absolute best.

This guide is divided into several sections, each about a different aspect of perimenopause, from the physical and emotional changes that occur during this phase to effective ways to manage symptoms. It also emphasizes the importance of self-care and how it can positively impact your overall well-being during perimenopause.

Additionally, this book explores the role of nutrition and exercise to support your body during this time, and will debunk common myths and misconceptions surrounding menopause. The goal is to provide you with a comprehensive understanding of perimenopause so that you can approach it with knowledge and confidence. And, if you are anything like me, you might want to take notes. So pages are included where you can document your journey, make notes on your symptoms and map out a plan of action to help you navigate the months and years ahead. Beyond just providing information, this workbook was designed to remind you that perimenopause can be a time for self-discovery and growth, an opportunity to prioritize your needs and desires, as well as rediscover your passions and purpose. I encourage you to embrace this new chapter of your life with open arms and a positive mindset.

I hope this guide serves as a valuable resource for you throughout your perimenopause journey. Remember, every woman's experience is unique, and what works for one may not work for another. Listen to your body; work with a medical provider that listens to your concerns and make informed decisions that align with your needs.

This information can support you every step of the way. I believe that with the right mindset and tools, you can navigate perimenopause gracefully and with confidence.

Thank you for including me on your journey. I wish you all the best in your perimenopause experience, as you keep learning, growing and thriving.

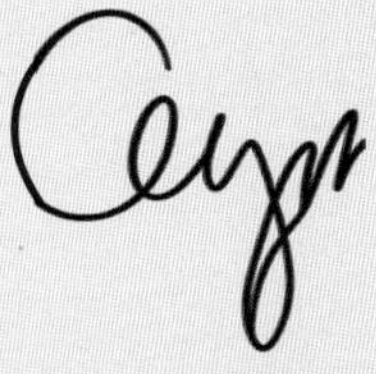

Chapter 1

Self Discovery

As I mentioned, perimenopause is not just about physical changes in the body, as it also marks a significant shift in your life that can bring new opportunities for self-discovery and personal growth. During this period, you have the chance to reflect on your past and present, re-evaluate your priorities and redefine goals.

Look how far you have come and decide how YOU want the rest of your life to play out. It's a time to let go of old patterns and beliefs that no longer serve you and embrace new perspectives and experiences.

Here are a few questions to help you consider where your journey is beginning.

What are 10 goals you want to accomplish in the next 5 years?

They can be personal or professional, physical or emotional. They can be big, sweeping changes or small, new habits that can be stacked to get you to these goals. Next to each big picture goal, jot down three small steps that will help you get there. Think "What can I do by the end of the month, and the end of the year?" and "What small steps can I start to implement to help me get there?"

1. __________
2. __________
3. __________
4. __________
5. __________
6. __________
7. __________
8. __________
9. __________
10. __________

What are you most proud of?

What are you most looking forward to?

1

What do you know now that you will take with you into this next phase of life?

What's a new yes you'd like to add to your life?

What is a belief that no longer serves you? Your body is telling you that big changes are coming,so why not take this as a sign to remove old thinking and habits?

One of the most important lessons you can learn during perimenopause is to prioritize your own needs and desires. as women, we often put others' needs before our own, but this phase of life is a reminder that self-care and self-love are crucial for our overall well-being. don't be afraid to say "no" to anything that drains your energy and focus on activities that bring you joy and fulfillment.

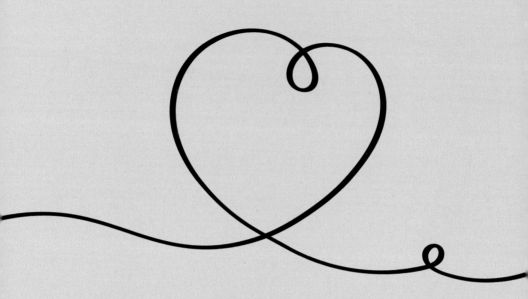

LOVE YOURSELF FIRST, AND EVERYTHING ELSE FALLS INTO LINE.

Lucille Ball

Self Care Checklist

- ☐ *Read a book*
- ☐ *Plan a fun day*
- ☐ *Cook your favorite meal*
- ☐ *Listen to music*
- ☐ *Take a nap*
- ☐ *Listen to a podcast*
- ☐ *Listen to an audiobook*
- ☐ *Watch a favorite movie*
- ☐ *Spend 10 min journaling*
- ☐ *Eat a healthy meal*
- ☐ *Go shopping*
- ☐ *Accomplish a goal*
- ☐ *Spend time outdoors*
- ☐ *Try something new*
- ☐ *Call your favorite person*
- ☐ *Create a vision board*
- ☐ *Take a bubble bath*
- ☐ *Go out with friends*
- ☐ *Learn something new*
- ☐ *Write yourself a love letter*
- ☐ *Buy yourself flowers*
- ☐ *Meditate*
- ☐ *Garden*
- ☐ *Go for a ride*
- ☐ *Go for a hike*
- ☐ *Go to the beach*
- ☐ *Drink a smoothie*
- ☐ *Plan a trip*
- ☐ *Go to a new city*
- ☐ *Write something*
- ☐ *Drink some tea*
- ☐ *Take a long shower*
- ☐ *Buy a new lotion*
- ☐ *Go to the gym*
- ☐ *Do what feels GOOD!*
- ☐ *Take a break from social media*

Chapter 2

The More You Know

The more you know about perimenopause, the better equipped you are to make informed decisions about your health and well-being. Take time to educate yourself on the physical, emotional and psychological changes that occur during this period. Talk to your doctor; read reliable sources of information; join support groups to connect with other women going through similar experiences.

Don't be afraid to reach out for support or hesitate to seek professional help as every woman needs to advocate for her health needs and have all the options that are available during this important transition.

Despite the challenges perimenopause may bring, you can use this time for growth and empowerment – especially with the right knowledge, support and mindset. You can embrace this phase of your life with confidence and positivity!

Start a menopause book club, join a Facebook group, listen to podcasts and make it a priority to support yourself and learn as much as you can during this time in your life.

Here is a list of incredible resources you can explore to give you extra knowledge.

- https://menopausefoundationcanada.ca
- https://www.mayoclinic.org/diseases-conditions/perimenopause/diagnosis treatment/drc-20354671
- https://www.canadianmenopausesociety.org/sites/default/files/pdf/publicati ons/Final-Pocket%20Guide.pdf
- www.mq6.ca
- MQ6 Menopause Management Tools
- Menopause Foundation of Canada, Menopause and U, Canadian Menopause Society GynQI - Understanding Menopause

Chapter 3

Are You In Perimenopause?

One of the most common questions I receive in my lectures is: "How do I know?"

Perimenopause generally begins for women in their 40s, although it can start as early as the mid-30s. The transitional phase leading up to menopause can last anywhere from several months to a decade, with an average duration of about four years. During perimenopause, the body's estrogen and progesterone production becomes irregular, which can result in various physical and emotional symptoms.

Recognizing the onset of perimenopause and understanding its effects is essential for managing this natural stage of life.

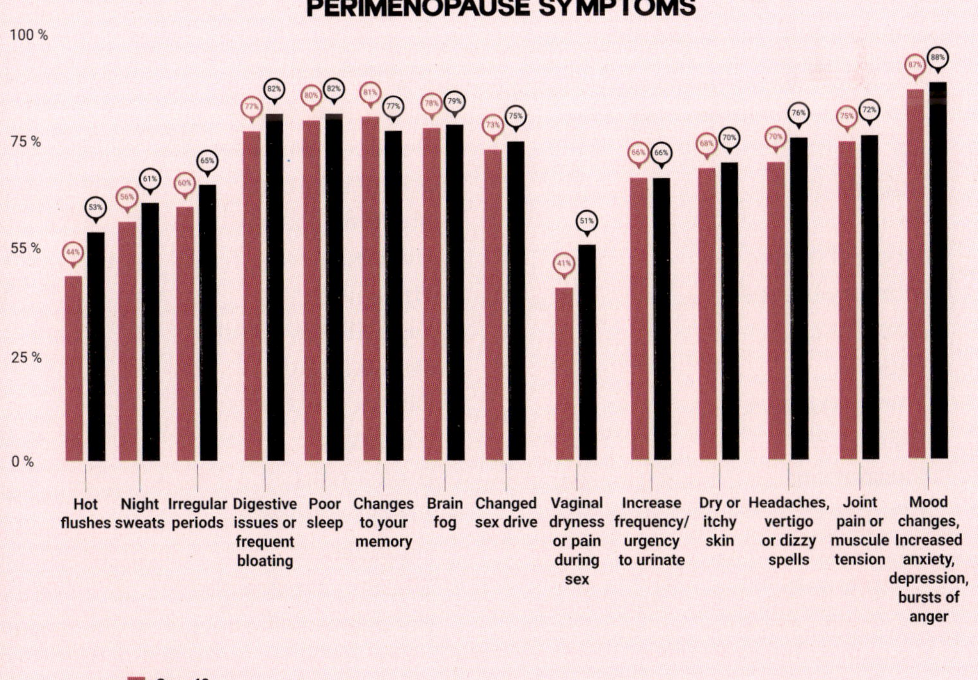

Common symptoms include irregular periods, anxiety, hot flashes, night sweats, mood swings, sleep issues, joint pain and changes in sexual desire. Some women may also experience cognitive changes, like forgetfulness or difficulty concentrating. All these symptoms are a normal part of the transition into menopause. They're not a disease or a disorder, but a natural phase of life.

Additionally, many women are asymptomatic and continue with a regular period; however, even if everything seems status quo, you can still be in perimenopause.

Menopause marks a significant transition in a woman's life, officially defined as occurring one year after her final period. This event can be a cause for celebration, as it signifies freedom from menstruation. Some women choose to commemorate it in unique ways, such as hosting parties.

Menopause Symptom List

- Hot flashes
- Anxiety
- Lack of concentration
- Irritability
- Panic
- Mood changes
- Memory lapses
- Depression
- Fatigue
- Thinning hair
- Brittle nails
- Palpitations
- Dizziness
- Body odor
- Weight gain
- Irregular periods
- Night sweats
- Disturbed sleep
- Reduced sex drive
- Vaginal dryness
- Muscle aches
- Bloating
- Nausea
- Digestion problems
- Dry, itchy skin
- Dental problems
- Joint pain
- Breast pain
- Breast changes
- Headaches
- Tingling extremities
- Bladder problems

Surgical menopause occurs the day the ovaries are surgically removed, a procedure known as an oophorectomy. This abrupt cessation of ovarian function can trigger immediate menopausal symptoms, making it vital to prepare in advance. If you are scheduled for this surgery, consulting with a hormone expert beforehand is essential to establish a hormone health plan that addresses your needs in the post-surgery period. It's important to note that a hysterectomy, which involves the removal of the uterus while leaving one or both ovaries intact, does not result in immediate menopause, as the ovaries continue to produce hormones for some time.

Postmenopause begins the day after the one-year anniversary of a woman's final menstrual period, marking a significant chapter in her life. This means adjusting to new norms for the rest of her life. During postmenopause, the body experiences a continuous decline in estrogen levels, which can lead to symptoms such as vaginal dryness and changes in mood or energy levels. Ensure that you stay informed about these changes and seek support for any discomforts that may arise, ensuring a healthier, more fulfilling postmenopausal life.

Developing a comprehensive health plan for the next several decades is vital, as hormonal fluctuations — including declining progesterone and estrogen — will impact overall well-being. Now is an ideal time to proactively explore strategies to support hormone health during this transformative period.

Track your changes. If you notice that certain symptoms progress from often to daily, for example, you may be inching ever closer to menopause. This will also help you narrow down the symptoms you're feeling (as opposed to just one, long, chaotic list of changes) and home in on the ones that are bothering you. This makes conversations with your doctor or naturopath more specific, allowing you both to develop a more targeted strategy to help deal with the most disruptive or uncomfortable symptoms.

Remember, the only constant throughout this process is change – meaning that this journey isn't linear, and things will fluctuate. But the more conscious you are of those fluctuations, the easier they will be to deal with as they wax and wane.

The following worksheets are not diagnostic but designed to help you recognize potential signs of perimenopause. If you answered "yes" to several of these questions and you're in your 40s or beyond, you may be entering perimenopause.

Please consult with a healthcare provider for a more accurate diagnosis. There is also more in the next chapter about how to talk to your healthcare provider(s) to create a plan for success.

Tracking symptoms makes conversations with your doctor more specific so you can create a targeted plan to deal with them.

Menopause Symptom Tracker

	HOW OFTEN I EXPERIENCE THIS SYMPTOM		
SYMPTOM	***NEVER***	***SOMETIMES***	***REGULARLY***
Hot Flashes			
Dizziness			
Night Sweats			
Disturbed Sleep			
Fatigue			
Palpitations			
Headaches			
Muscle aches			
Joint Pain			
Thinning Hair			
Breast Changes			
Weight Gain			
Dry and Itchy Skin			
Reduced Sex Drive			
Vaginal Dryness			
Irregular Periods			
Mood Changes			
Anxiety Concentration			
Lack of Concentration			
Memory Lapses			

Menopause Symptom Tracker

SYMPTOM BEING TRACKED:	
WEEK BEGINNING DATE:	

	MORNING	AFTERNOON	EVENING	NIGHT
MON				
TUE				
WED				
THU				
FRI				
SAT				
SUN				

MORNING

MONTH: ______________________

	1	2	3	4	5	6	7	8	9	10	11	12	13	14	15	16	17	18	19	20	21	22	23	24	25	26	27	28	29	30	31
Hot Flashes																															
Dizziness																															
Night Sweats																															
Disturbed Sleep																															
Fatigue																															
Palpitations																															
Headaches																															
Muscle aches																															
Joint Pain																															
Thinning Hair																															
Breast Changes																															
Weight Gain																															
Dry, Itchy Skin																															
Low Sex Drive																															
Vaginal Dryness																															
Irregular Periods																															
Mood Changes																															
Anxiety																															
Concentration																															
Memory Lapses																															

Chapter 4

The Menopause Plan

Just as expecting mothers develop a birthing plan, women should prepare a comprehensive menopause plan well in advance,to address symptoms, health risks and potential treatments. Further, approaching this significant transition with a plan will help you maintain your health and well-being.

Open, honest conversations with healthcare providers can help you navigate this stage and create an effective path. Here are important topics to discuss.

Understanding Menopause

Begin by asking your doctor for a thorough explanation of what menopause is, the stages involved and what symptoms to expect. Knowledge is power, and understanding the process can alleviate anxiety.

Symptoms Management

Discuss the symptoms you're experiencing or might expect, from hot flashes and night sweats to mood swings and bone density loss. Ask about lifestyle changes or treatments available to manage these symptoms effectively.

Menopause Hormone Therapy

Inquire about the risks and benefits of MHT. Discuss whether it is beneficial for you or if there are alternative therapies you should consider.

Long-Term Health Implications

Menopause can have long-term effects on heart health, bone density and more. Ask your doctor about ways to mitigate these risks through diet, exercise, supplementation or medication.

Mental Health Support

Ask what support options, including counseling and support groups, are available to help manage emotional changes and challenges.

Regular Screenings & Tests

Find out what routine health screenings you should continue or start as you transition through menopause, such as mammograms, bone density tests and cholesterol checks.

Lifestyle Changes

Request information about lifestyle changes that can aid in a smoother transition, such as dietary adjustments, exercise routines and stress management techniques.

Specific Questions to Ask Your Medical Provider:

1. What are the common symptoms? Which am I most likely to experience?
2. How can I differentiate between menopause symptoms and other health issues?
3. Are there lifestyle changes I should adopt now to ease symptoms and improve health outcomes?
4. What are the pros and cons of menopause hormone therapy for someone with my health profile?
5. How can menopause impact my mental health? What resources are available to help?
6. Which regular screenings should I prioritize during and after menopause?
7. What supplements or vitamins do you recommend to ensure I maintain good health?
8. How often should we meet to discuss my menopause plan and make necessary adjustments?

By preparing for your discussions with these questions and topics in mind, you can ensure a proactive approach to managing your mid-life hormonal care effectively.

I f you are looking for a practitioner in your area or online, Aeyron Wellness has an incredible resource available of more than 400 health practitioners all across Canada on our website:

www.aeryonwellness.com/practioner.

Navigating menopause is a highly personal experience, and finding the right health practitioner to guide you through it can make a significant difference. Choose someone who respects your concerns and aligns with your health goals.

A practitioner who fearmongers or dismisses or questions your symptoms, can undermine your confidence and hinder effective healthcare management. In such cases, it is imperative to seek a second opinion or find a healthcare provider who listens, supports and collaborates with you.

Your health journey deserves a compassionate partner who acknowledges your experiences and empowers you to make informed decisions.

Bring a pen and take notes at your appointment, record the conversation with your doctor on your phone, or, if you're comfortable, bring a friend or family member to take the notes for you. Often, these appointments can feel rushed, and you may not feel like you're absorbing all of the information, so being able to reference it back can be helpful.

Consider booking a follow-up appointment to go over some of the information and ask follow-up questions. As discussed in Chapter 3, some of your symptoms and their severity can change with time. You're your best advocate; you know your body; and your doctor is only able to work with what you tell her. Be specific, bring notes and keep track of all of it. It may sound daunting and like one more thing on your to-do list, but it will take you less than five minutes a day once you get in the habit, and this data can really help.

Chapter 5

Hormones And Perimenopause

Hormones are tiny chemical messengers throughout the body that, though small, play a crucial role in regulating numerous bodily functions. Produced by glands in the endocrine system and released into the bloodstream, they travel to various tissues and organs to exert their effects.

Endocrine Glands and Major Hormones

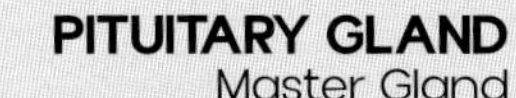

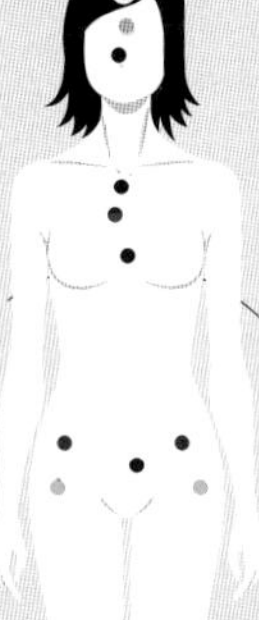

PITUITARY GLAND
Master Gland
Secretes hormones that control other glands

ENDOCRINE GLANDS AND MAJOR HORMONES
Governor of the Endocrine System
Controls the pituitary gland

OTHER ENCOCRINE GLANDS
Pinal Gland, Thyriod & Parathyroid, Thymus, Pancreas

ADRENAL GLANDS
Produces testosterone (in small amounts) that helps with sexual responce

OVARIES
Produces estrogen that controls mentruation &progesterone that supports pregnency

The hormonal feedback loop is a system of checks and balances, ensuring that hormone levels remain within an optimal range. This loop involves three main components:

1. A stimulus that triggers hormone release;
2. The gland's response to the stimulus by either increasing or decreasing hormone secretion;
3. The effect of the hormone on the target organ that ultimately feeds back to the gland, signaling to maintain or alter production.

5

Through this mechanism, the body maintains homeostasis, such as regulating metabolism, growth, mood and reproductive processes, highlighting the complexity and sophistication of hormonal interactions. As you go through perimenopause, this homeostasis is disrupted and, though these hormones are small, they can have huge effects in your overall health and well-being.

A woman's body features several key hormones that play crucial roles in various physiological processes. The main ones during perimenopause include estrogen, progesterone and testosterone. During this time, production of these hormones begins to fluctuate and decrease as previously mentioned. This phase can last for several years and typically begins in a woman's late 30s to 40s, although it can start earlier.

Chapter 6

The Roles Of Hormones

Estrogen is a vital hormone that influences numerous physiological processes throughout a woman's life, primarily in regulating the menstrual cycle and maintaining reproductive health. In addition to its reproductive functions, estrogen plays a significant role in promoting healthy skin, maintaining bone density and supporting cardiovascular health. This hormone is primarily produced in the ovaries, though smaller amounts are also made in the adrenal glands and fat cells.

Estrogen levels fluctuate throughout a woman's menstrual cycle, with the highest concentrations just before ovulation (the follicular phase), and a sharp drop afterward if pregnancy doesn't occur. The production of estrogen is controlled by the pituitary gland, which releases Follicle Stimulating Hormone (FSH) and Luteinizing Hormone (LH) to trigger the production and release of estrogen.

However, as women transition through perimenopause and menopause, fluctuations and declines in estrogen levels can lead to various symptoms and health concerns that require careful management and support. During perimenopause, the levels of estrogen can often be 20 to 30% higher and sporadic, which can be defined as "hormonal chaos." Often marked by irregular menstrual cycles, this period can start several years before menopause.

Indications of changing estrogen levels during perimenopause may include hot flashes, night sweats, mood swings, sleep disturbances, vaginal dryness and irregular periods. Each woman's experience may differ and depend on genetics and lifestyle causing symptoms to range from mild to severe

FLUCTUATIONS IN ESTRODIAL AND PROGESTERONE

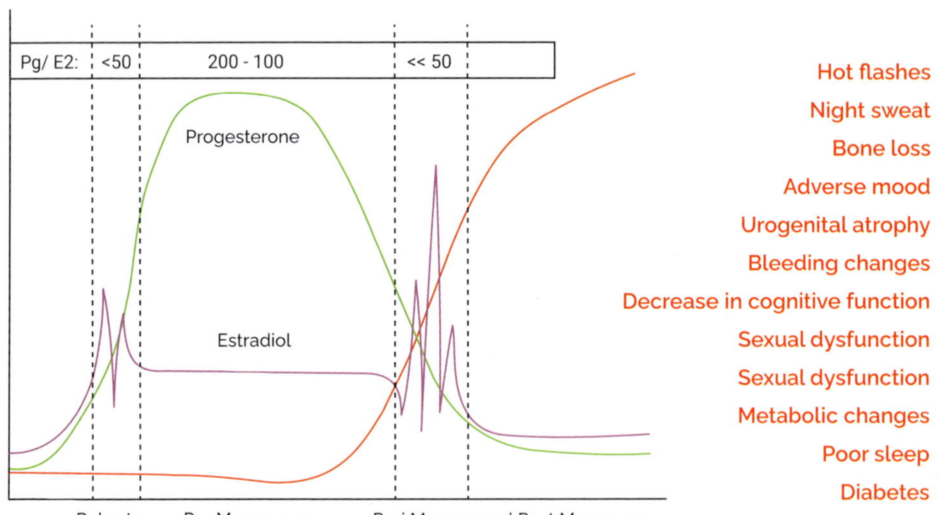

Changes or decreases in estrogen levels can lead to several challenges, including:

- Episodes of hot flashes or night sweats
- Memory issues
- Dryness of the vulva/vagina
- Discomfort during intercourse
- Increased susceptibility to urinary tract infections (UTIs)
- Urinary incontinence
- Pelvic organ prolapse
- Reduced libido
- Joint discomfort
- Dryness in the eyes, mouth, hair and skin

After menopause, the ovaries stop producing significant amounts of estrogen, resulting in much lower levels of this crucial hormone. While this hormonal shift is natural and expected, it can have noticeable effects on a woman's health and well-being. Lower estrogen levels are associated with symptoms such as vaginal dryness, reduced bone density and increased risk of cardiovascular issues.

However, this phase is also an opportunity to focus on strategies that support long-term health.

Understanding the changes that occur after menopause is empowering. By maintaining a balanced diet rich in calcium and vitamin D, engaging in regular weight-bearing exercises and exploring medical options such as menopause hormone therapy (MHT) when appropriate, women can take charge of their health.

While the decline in estrogen may bring challenges, it may also offer you a time to thrive with intention, care and confidence. This stage signifies resilience and an opportunity to prioritize one's well-being and strength.

ESTROGEN HORMONE LEVEL

MENOPAUSE

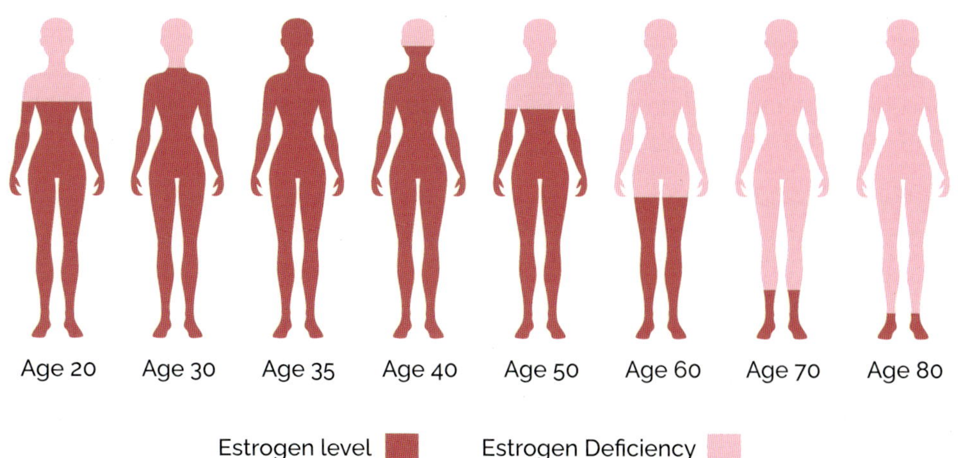

Estrogen

Progesterone

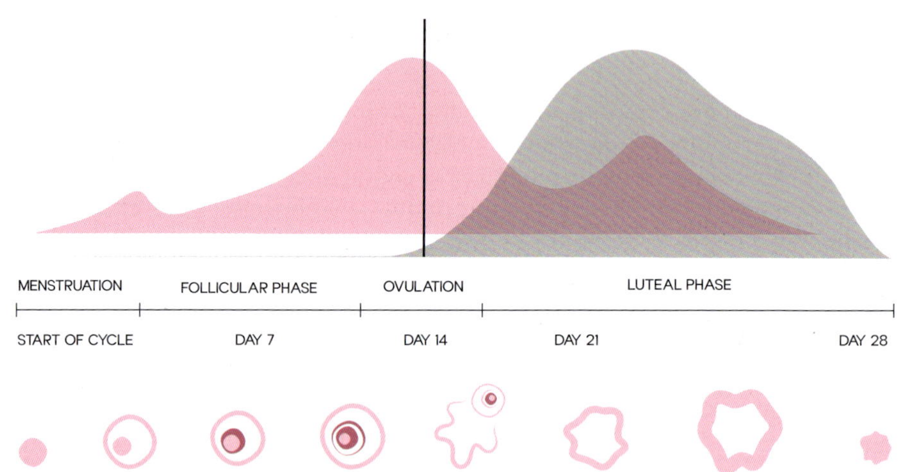

Progesterone is an endogenous steroid hormone predominantly produced by the ovaries and the adrenals. During the initial 10 weeks of pregnancy, the ovarian corpus luteum secretes progesterone, after which the placenta takes over its production. When pregnancy does not occur, progesterone levels drop drastically as the corpus luteum degenerates, a process known as luteolysis. The reduced progesterone level leads to the shedding of the uterine lining, resulting in menstrual bleeding.

This hormone not only helps regulate the menstrual cycle and maintain a healthy uterus but also plays an important role in mood stabilization and sleep quality.

During perimenopause, one of the primary changes involves a decrease in progesterone levels. This decline occurs because ovulation becomes less frequent and eventually ceases altogether as the ovaries age and their functionality declines. Since progesterone is primarily produced by the corpus luteum following ovulation, less frequent ovulation leads to lower progesterone production.

This hormonal shift can contribute to symptoms often associated with perimenopause, such as irregular menstrual cycles, sleep disturbances and mood swings. Understanding these hormonal changes is crucial for managing the symptoms and preparing for the eventual onset of menopause.

Managing progesterone levels effectively, either through lifestyle choices, supplements like Reclaim Hormonal Support from Aeryon Wellness, or medical interventions, can be supportive during perimenopause. Restoring hormonal balance can mitigate the symptoms of perimenopause and enhance your overall well-being during this transition.

Variations or reductions in progesterone levels may lead to:

- Trouble focusing
- Emotional ups and downs
- Feelings of sadness
- Heightened anxiety
- Migraines
- Trouble sleeping
- Tenderness or swelling in the breasts
- Sudden heat sensations
- Bloating
- Premenstrual syndrome (PMS)
- Night sweats or hot flashes
- Heavy or unpredictable menstrual bleeding

Testosterone often regarded as a male hormone, plays an essential role in women's health, influencing both physical and emotional well-being. It contributes to a woman's energy levels, mood, cognitive function and sexual drive. Reduced testosterone levels during perimenopause can lead to lowered vitality and sexual interest, which can affect a woman's quality of life.

Furthermore, testosterone plays a crucial role in bone health. Lower levels are linked to a higher risk of osteoporosis, a condition that becomes more prevalent as women transition into menopause. Therefore, maintaining balanced testosterone levels can be as important as managing the levels of estrogen and progesterone during perimenopause. When testosterone levels fluctuate or decline, women may face a range of challenges, including decreased sexual desire, low energy, diminished motivation and heightened feelings of emotional disconnect.

Proper hormonal balance can alleviate the symptoms of perimenopause, enhancing a woman's overall well-being during this life transition

Variations or reductions in testosterone levels may lead to several challenges, including:

- Decreased libido
- Lack of drive
- Low energy or mood
- Reduced sense of well-being
- Muted emotional responses
- Diminished self-confidence
- Lack of muscle

Cortisol often referred to as the stress hormone, helps regulate various bodily functions, especially during perimenopause and menopause. Elevated cortisol levels contribute to fatigue and weight gain, particularly around the waist, while low levels may leave women feeling drained and lethargic. Understanding cortisol's impact is essential for addressing women's health concerns, as imbalances can disrupt sleep, sexual health and overall wellness.

Beyond the obvious feelings of fatigue and weight gain, these effects can compound the challenges many women face during perimenopause. Managing stress through lifestyle changes, mindfulness practices and regular exercise can mitigate elevated cortisol levels. Supplementing, specifically with U Got This Stress Support, can offer a smoother transition, promoting overall hormonal balance.

Fluctuations in cortisol levels can lead to a variety of challenges, such as:

- Heightened stress
- Feeling exhausted yet restless
- Difficulty sleeping
- Increased irritability
- Episodes of dizziness
- Anxiety
- Feelings of depression
- Weight gain, particularly around the waist
- Persistent fatigue
- Intense cravings for food
- Bodily aches and pains
- Greater frequency of colds or flu
- Exacerbation of chronic conditions, including diabetes

The thyroid is a butterfly-shaped gland in the neck that plays a pivotal role in regulating metabolism, energy production and overall hormonal balance. It produces several key hormones, including TSH (Thyroid Stimulating Hormone), T4 (Thyroxine) and T3 (Triiodothyronine), which work in concert to ensure that the body's systems function optimally. When the thyroid is functioning properly, individuals often experience heightened energy levels and improved mood; however, both hypothyroidism and hyperthyroidism can lead to significant health challenges that warrant attention and support.

Perimenopause can significantly affect thyroid function due to the fluctuations in hormone levels that occur during this transitional phase.

As estrogen and progesterone levels vary, they can influence the production and regulation of thyroid hormones, leading to potential imbalances. Many women may experience symptoms such as fatigue, weight gain and mood swings, which thyroid dysfunction can exacerbate.

Furthermore, the thyroid may become more sensitive to the hormonal changes brought on by perimenopause, which means women need to monitor their thyroid health during this time.

If you experience unusual fatigue, weight gain, dry skin, menstrual irregularities or cold intolerance, have your thyroid hormones checked. Hypothyroidism, characterized by an under-functioning thyroid gland, is one of the most common thyroid conditions. Hashimoto's thyroiditis is a prevalent form of hypothyroidism, is autoimmune in nature and occurs when the body's immune system attacks the thyroid gland causing inflammation and reduced thyroid function.

Hashimoto's thyroiditis primarily affects women. Symptoms can include fatigue, constipation, dry skin, weight gain, cold intolerance, voice hoarseness, slowed movements, memory loss, joint pains, hair loss, menstrual irregularities and depression. Diagnosis involves physical examination findings and blood tests to measure thyroid hormone levels and specific antibodies associated with the autoimmune process.

Understanding and addressing the underlying autoimmune process helps you reduce the risk of developing autoimmune conditions and promote optimal thyroid health. Regular screenings are essential, especially if you have a family history of autoimmune thyroid or other autoimmune diseases. A comprehensive approach to managing Hashimoto's thyroiditis allows for a more holistic and personalized treatment plan, targeting the root cause and supporting long-term health.

Addressing thyroid imbalances can alleviate some of the symptoms associated with perimenopause, ultimately improving overall quality of life.

Variations in thyroid hormone levels can lead to several issues, including:

- **Persistent tiredness**
- **Sensation of cold in the extremities**
- **Reduced body temperature**
- **Difficulty shedding pounds**
- **Irregular bowel movements**
- **Feelings of sadness or depression**
- **Dry and flaky skin**
- **Brittle nails and hair loss**
- **Difficulties with focus and attention**
- **Muscle discomfort**
- **Swelling around the eyes and face**
- **Decreased interest in sexual activity**

HORMONE NAME	WHAT IS IT?	WHERE IS IT MADE?	WHAT DOES IT DO?
Estradiol (Estrogen) aka: E2 estradiol - 1 7β-estradiol	- Strongest of the three types of estrogen - A steroid hormone made from cholesterol	- Mostly in the ovaries - Smaller amounts in other tissues such as the brain, fat tissue, and blood vessel walls	- Primary activity is with the reproductive system - Maintains and controls the menstrual cycle - Triggers breast tissue development - Increases bone and cartilage density - Acts on multiple centers in the brain
Estrone (Estrogen) aka: E1 - oestron	- Weaker form of estrogen - Major type of estrogen produced post-menopause	- Mostly in the ovaries - Some from the adrenal gland - Smaller amounts from fat tissue	- Specifics are poorly understood - As an estrogen, it is involved in the female reproductive system
Estriol (Estrogen) aka: E3 - oestriol	- Exists in very low levels in non-pregnant women	- High amounts produced by the placenta - Triggered by a chemical produced in the fetus' adrenal gland	- Involved in uterine growth - Helps prepare the body for childbirth
Progesterone	- Member of a group of steroid hormones called progestogens	- In the corpus luteum in the ovaries. The corpus luteum is formed from a ruptured follicle that just released an egg	- Causes the lining of the uterus to thicken in preparation for pregnancy after an egg is released - If there is no pregnancy, the corpus luteum (where the progesterone is formed) breaks down, dropping progesterone levels and triggering menstruation
Testosterone aka: -4-androsten-17β-o-3-one	- Member (and best known) of a group of hormones called androgens	- Mostly in the adrenal gland - Small amounts in the ovaries	- Stimulates development of male characteristics - Enhances libido
Follicle-stimulating Hormone (FSH)	- Member of a group of hormones called gonadotropins	- The anterior pituitary gland (from cells called gonadotrophs) - Its release is regulated by the hypothalamus	- Essential for development at puberty - Triggers the release of estrogen - Triggers egg development
Luteinising hormone (LH)	- Member of a group of hormones called gonadotropins	- The anterior pituitary gland (from cells called gonadotrophs) - Release is regulated by the hypothalamus	- Triggers ovulation (the release of an egg) - Triggers estrogen and progesterone production from the corpus luteum

Hormonal Cheat Sheet

ESTROGEN: The main function is to prepare the female reproductive system to make it fertile. It also affects hair growth, body fat, bone health, vaginal health, cognition, sleep, collagen production, and more.

ESTRADIOL (E2): Primary form of estrogen during reproductive years, the most potent.

ESTRIOL (E3): The primary form of estrogen when pregnant.

ESTRONE (E1): Primary form of estrogen after menopause.

PROGESTERONE: The main role is to prepare the uterus lining to receive the fertilized egg; however, it also helps balance estrogen.

FSH: Stimulates follicles on the ovary to grow and prepare the eggs for ovulation.

LH: Helps control the menstrual cycle. It also triggers the release of an egg from the ovary.

TESTOSTERONE: Influences libido, bone health, regulation of the menstrual cycle, and muscle.

CORTISOL: Assists our body in response to stress.

Chapter 7

Your Monthly Report Card

Experiencing severe symptoms during premenstrual syndrome (PMS) is not standard or healthy. Rather than accepting intense discomfort as a normal part of the menstrual cycle, it is more constructive to view our periods as monthly health "report cards." They provide valuable insights into our overall well-being and hormonal balance. A well-regulated and smooth menstrual cycle is indicative of optimal hormone functioning, which not only improves quality of life but also paves the way for a more seamless transition into menopause later in life. By addressing and managing menstrual irregularities, women can foster long-term hormonal health and mitigate potential issues associated with hormonal changes as they age.

One of the best ways to understand how your hormones are functioning is to collect data. This period tracker will allow you to see what is happening with your cycle and record any specific details that will be helpful for you and your medical professional. Beyond just the length of your cycle, you can keep track of things like the volume of blood, your mood, appetite, energy levels and more.

All of these are important factors in analyzing the overall status of your hormones. Online tracking apps are also helpful in documenting the changes from month to month.

Hormonal imbalance can be a reason why PMS occurs. An excess or deficiency in the production of hormones can lead to disruptions in the body's normal functioning. This imbalance can manifest through a variety of symptoms, such as fatigue, mood swings, weight fluctuations and changes in appetite or sleep patterns. Various factors can contribute to hormonal imbalances, including stress, poor diet, medical conditions like polycystic ovary syndrome or thyroid disorders and lifestyle habits.

Additionally, exposure to external substances known as xenoestrogens can exacerbate hormonal disruptions. Xenoestrogens are synthetic compounds found in pesticides, plastics, personal care products and certain foods that mimic the action of estrogen in the body, potentially altering natural hormone levels creating estrogen excess. Xenoestrogens, chemically similar to natural estrogen, can bind to estrogen receptors in the body, intensifying the effects of estrogen and leading to an array of symptoms associated with estrogen excess.

Eliminating exposure to xenoestrogens can also significantly support perimenopause management. This proactive approach not only alleviates potential symptoms associated with estrogen dominance, such as hot flashes and mood swings, but also fosters a smoother perimenopausal experience overall.

Implementing lifestyle changes, such as choosing organic produce, using natural household products and avoiding plastic containers, can be effective strategies in reducing xenoestrogen exposure and promoting hormonal health.

Additionally, supporting our liver in metabolizing excess estrogen is crucial for maintaining hormonal balance and overall health. The liver plays a vital role in detoxifying the body by breaking down and excreting excess hormones, including estrogen. When the liver functions efficiently, it processes estrogen into its metabolizable form, which is then eliminated from the body. However, if the liver is overburdened due to poor diet, exposure to environmental toxins or excessive alcohol consumption, it can struggle to metabolize estrogen effectively, which can lead to an accumulation of estrogen and contribute to the symptoms associated with estrogen dominance.

Therefore, supporting liver health through a balanced diet rich in cruciferous vegetables, maintaining adequate hydration, and avoiding excessive intake of alcohol and processed foods can significantly enhance its ability to metabolize estrogen and thereby promote hormonal equilibrium and reduce the risk of associated health issues.

Functions of the healthy liver

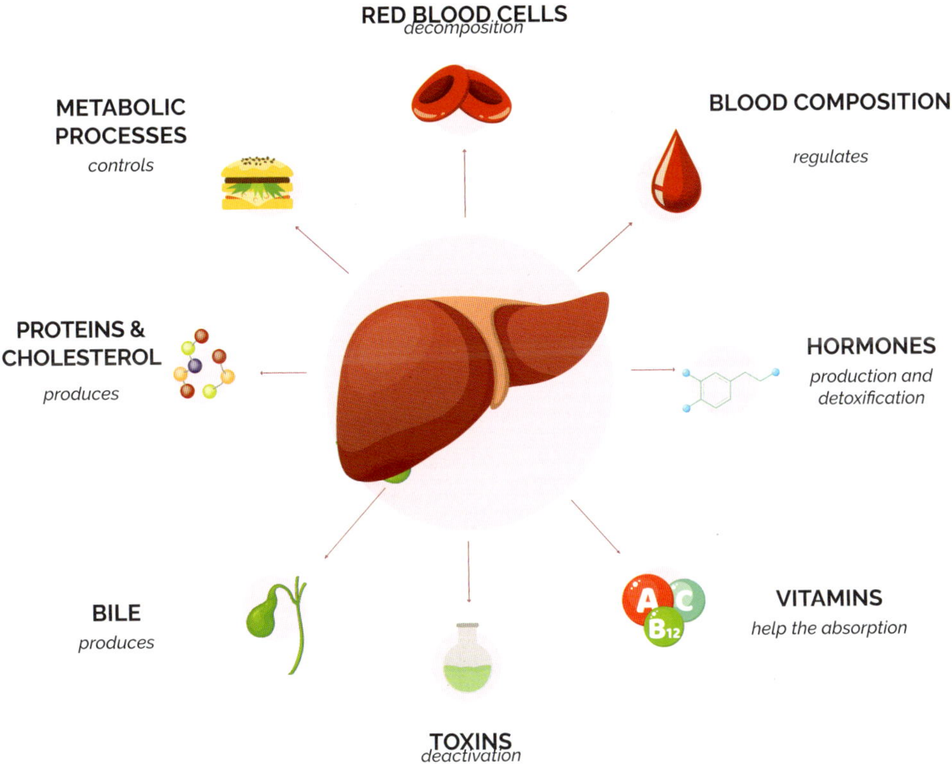

Hormonal imbalance can be a reason why pms occurs; an excess or deficiency in the production of hormones can lead to disruptions in the body's normal functioning.

Period Tracker

	JAN	FEB	MAR	APR	MAY	JUN	JUL	AUG	SEP	OCT	NOV	DEC
1												
2												
3												
4												
5												
6												
7												
8												
9												
10												
11												
12												
13												
14												
15												
16												
17												
18												
19												
20												
21												
22												
23												
24												
25												
26												
27												
28												
29												
30												
31												

KEY	

CYCLE LENGTH	
JANUARY	
FEBRUARY	
MARCH	
APRIL	
MAY	
JUNE	
JULY	
AUGUST	
SEPTEMBER	
OCTOBER	
NOVEMBER	
DECEMBER	

NOTES

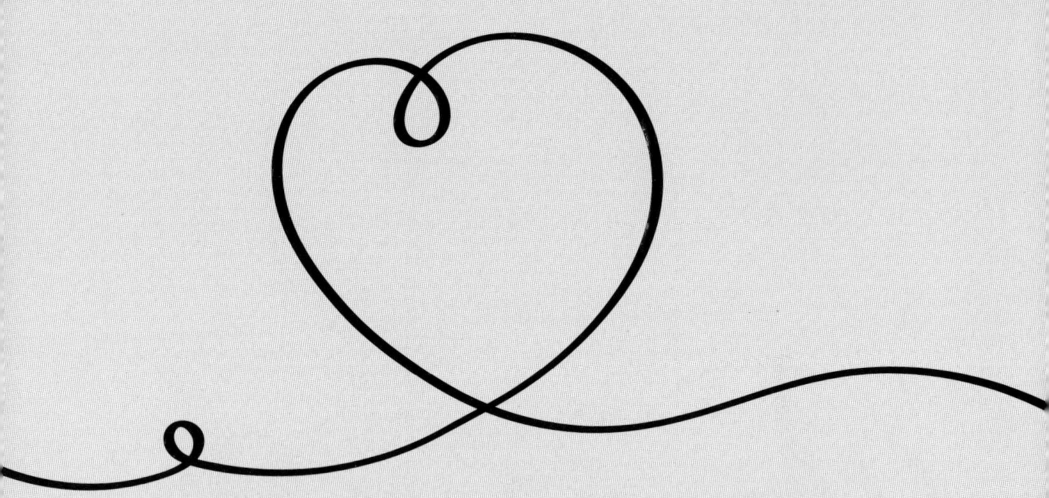

EVERY PERIOD
IS A CHANCE TO
CELEBRATE YOUR
BODY'S POWER

Chapter 8

Hormone Testing

Tracking your hormone levels over the years can be eye-opening to help understand what is happening to your body. I started blood panels at 35 when my hormones were all over the place, then I proceeded to test once every five years. I wanted to be proactive with all the information at hand as I approached midlife. A variety of tests are available to monitor hormone levels, each offering unique insights.

During perimenopause, estrogen levels typically fluctuate and can be inconsistent, sometimes high and other times low. Progesterone levels can decrease during this period. Additionally, elevations in FSH, a hormone responsible for stimulating the growth of the ovarian follicle, are commonly observed. Furthermore, LH, which stimulates the release of the egg during ovulation, can fluctuate significantly. It's worth noting that these changes can vary greatly from woman to woman, and the presence of symptoms often plays a key role in diagnosing perimenopause along with these hormonal shifts. Your healthcare practitioner will often refer to these tests when looking at your hormonal care plan.

Blood tests are commonly recommended, as they measure levels of estrogen, progesterone, FSH and LH. These hormones are key players in the menstrual cycle, can fluctuate throughout perimenopause and be measured through your family physician. These are free Canada; however, many women have shared their frustration with being dismissed or told they cannot have these tests by their MDs. Please read ***Chapter Four*** on how to approach your doctor to advocate for your midlife care.

Another useful tool for tracking hormone levels is the DUTCH test (Dried Urine Test for Comprehensive Hormones). This innovative testing method measures key sex hormones and their metabolites via dried urine samples collected at four points throughout the day. The DUTCH test provides a comprehensive view of your hormone levels and can provide valuable insights into hormone imbalances that could be contributing to perimenopause symptoms. This test costs roughly $500, though is often covered by extended benefits and ordered through a Naturopathic Doctor.

Hormone level tests provide you the opportunity to get curious about your body and understand what is happening. I firmly support women at any age asking for testing if they are not feeling well, as it provides valuable information for your healthcare provider to make informed decisions about your treatment plan and puts you in the driver seat of your health and wellness journey.

For ovarian reserve, you would test in the luteal phase or the 21st day of your cycle. If you are testing for fertility, testing in the follicular phase, which is after your menstrual cycle. If you no longer have a cycle due to medical intervention you can use a thermometer to check vaginal temperature as you should be the highest during ovulation.

01

Bone Density Test (DEXA Scan)

Given the increased risk of osteoporosis post-menopause, a bone density test helps assess bone mineral loss and the risk of fractures, enabling timely intervention.

02

Lipid Profile

As cardiovascular risk increases during menopause, a lipid profile can help monitor cholesterol levels, ensuring steps can be taken to maintain heart health.

03

Thyroid Function Test

With thyroid issues being common to emerge during perimenopause, testing for hormone levels like TSH, T3 and T 4 can detect any dysfunction early.

04

Blood Sugar Level

Considering metabolic changes that can accompany menopause, checking blood glucose levels can aid in the early detection and management of diabetes or insulin resistance. DEXCOM is a great over-the-counter option to start checking your blood sugar levels.

Work with a health practitioner or a team of practitioners to help you listen to your symptoms and decide the best form of treatment for you. Find a health practitioner in your area at

www.aeryonwellness.com/practioners.

Chapter 9

Reducing The Risks

Midlife presents a unique and often challenging chapter in a woman's life, where health concerns — both immediate and long-term — demand your attention like never before. Many of us start to feel the pressing weight of statistics and warnings about heart disease, osteoporosis, dementia and other conditions that disproportionately affect women. Yet, these years also offer an incredible opportunity, a chance to shift the narrative, take control and prioritize your well-being to strengthen your present and future self.

The choices you make now will shape the vitality of your heart, mind, bone and more in the years ahead. This chapter is about empowerment, education and action, because your health is worth the investment, starting today.

HEART HEALTH

Our risk of dying from heart disease is seven times higher than dying from breast cancer. This staggering statistic underscores the critical importance of prioritizing heart health now. By evaluating key lifestyle factors, such as how you eat, move, sleep and manage stress, you can address any gaps in nutritional support and open a dialogue with your health care team to set personalized heart health goals.

Understanding your risk factors is crucial. For instance, women with a history of endometriosis, polycystic ovarian syndrome, gestational diabetes or high blood pressure during pregnancy may face a higher risk of cardiovascular disease.

You also can shift your perspective on the symptoms of hormonal changes, such as hot flashes or night sweats. Rather than seeing these as mere nuisances, you can view them as a chance to prioritize self-care—like putting your own oxygen mask on first. These signals from your body are a call to action, urging you to respond with informed and proactive measures. By doing so, you can take meaningful steps to protect your heart health and address the pressing cardiovascular challenges that many women face as they age.

BONE HEALTH AND OSTEOPOROSIS

Talking about bone health is not easy, as it's a topic that often takes a backseat in conversations about women's health. However, the reality is that osteoporosis and its associated risks demand attention. The statistics are sobering, with fractures leading to serious consequences such as reduced mobility, loss of independence and even potential links to dementia. For women, particularly those approaching menopause or experiencing early menopause, the stakes are even higher. Lower estrogen levels during this stage significantly impact bone density, increasing the risk of fractures.

If you find yourself wishing for your period to stop, remember that its continuation can offer protective benefits to your bone health. Estrogen plays a critical role in maintaining bone density, making hormone balance essential for healthy bones.

Bone is more than just structural support; it's a dynamic, living tissue that contributes to overall health. For example, the hormone osteocalcin, produced in the bones, influences the Hypothalamus-Pituitary-Adrenal (HPA) axis, which is central to the body's stress response. Osteocalcin also regulates metabolism, reproduction and cognition. It increases insulin production and secretion, and increases the sensitivity of skeletal muscle and adipose tissue to insulin.

Lifestyle choices are equally powerful in protecting and strengthening your bones. Incorporating strength-building and jump-training exercises into your daily routine can help increase bone density and lean muscle mass. Reducing alcohol consumption and not smoking are also vital to prevent bone deterioration.

Nutrition is another key factor. Ensure adequate intake of calcium, vitamin D and other critical nutrients like magnesium, vitamins D3/K2, and omega-3s. These supplements, when combined with a balanced diet and regular exercise, enhance bone density and strength.

Consult with your doctor about your bone health, particularly if you have underlying health conditions such as arthritis, diabetes or thyroid disease. Discuss whether hormone therapy can provide benefits for preventing osteoporosis and take advantage of professional guidance to address your individual needs. With increased awareness, lifestyle adjustments and proactive measures, you can mitigate the impact of bone-related risks, empowering yourself for a stronger, healthier and more resilient future.

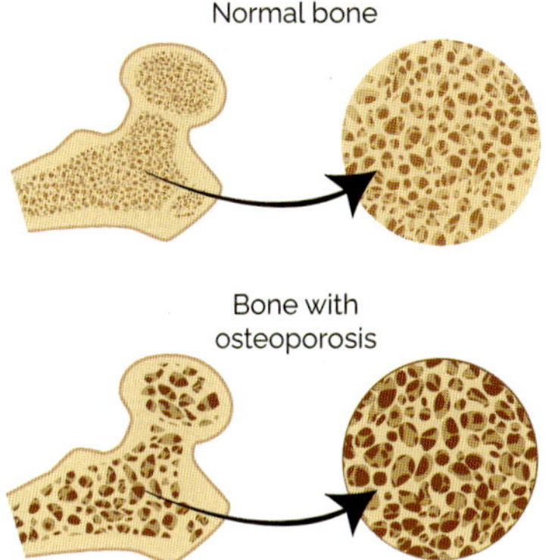

ESTROGEN PLAYS A CRITICAL ROLE IN MAINTAINING BONE DENSITY, MAKING HORMONE BALANCE ESSENTIAL FOR HEALTHY BINES.

INSULIN RESISTANCE

Insulin resistance is a significant concern for middle-aged women, particularly during the early stages of perimenopause when hormonal fluctuations lead to metabolic changes and are often exacerbated by the additional activity of fat cells acting as mini estrogen factories. This not only promotes weight gain but also contributes to an estrogen excess that triggers numerous symptoms. Women nearing menopause become particularly vulnerable to insulin resistance because of increasing fat mass and a gradual reduction in muscle mass, which decreases the body's ability to regulate blood sugar effectively .

To manage insulin resistance, adopt targeted lifestyle strategies, like increasing protein intake. Aim for 30 grams of high-quality protein per meal to help build and maintain muscle mass, which naturally burns more calories than fat. Consuming foods with a low glycemic index supports stable blood sugar levels by avoiding sharp spikes. Incorporate at least 25 grams of dietary fibre daily to promote better blood sugar balance and support gut health. Additionally, including healthy fats from sources such as avocados, fatty fish and nuts aids in maintaining proper hormone production and metabolic function. Balancing meals to include proteins, healthy fats and complex carbohydrates ensures consistent energy levels and supports metabolic efficiency. Establishing a habit of eating a nutritious breakfast daily can also kickstart metabolism and set a positive tone for managing blood sugar throughout the day. Finally, including blood sugar support supplements like So Hormonious is clinically proven to support blood sugar and hormone balance.

Emerging clinical data highlights the critical role of these dietary and lifestyle interventions in reducing the risk of insulin resistance. Studies emphasize that even modest improvements in muscle mass and reductions in visceral fat can significantly improve insulin sensitivity. Regular exercise combined with these nutritional adjustments has been shown to improve metabolic markers, stabilize glucose levels and boost overall energy. By understanding the interplay between metabolic changes, diet and lifestyle, women in this life stage can proactively take control of their health, minimizing the risk of insulin resistance and associated complications such as Type 2 diabetes.

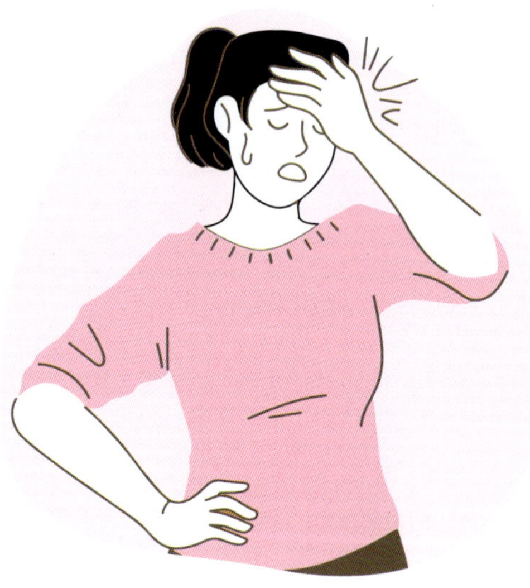

SYMPTOMS OF INSULIN RESISTANCE

	Abdominal obesity
	Difficulty losing weight
	Craving for sugar or carbohydrate-rich foods
	Fatty Liver
	Chronic fatigue or low energy
	Brain fog
	High blood sugar levels
	Skin tags
	Dark patches on the skin
	High blood pressure
	Frequent urination
	Thirsty all the time

Menopause Fact

60% of middle-aged women
report difficulty concentrating and other issues with cognition. These issues spike in women going through perimenopause.

BRAIN HEALTH

Brain health is pivotal in maintaining overall well-being, especially during hormonally dynamic periods like menopause. During this stage, the brain experiences a shift in energy utilization and metabolic activity, necessitating proactive measures to protect cognitive function and reduce the risk of long-term neurodegenerative conditions. You can support brain health through a combination of targeted lifestyle adjustments and mindful interventions. Maintaining an active, physical lifestyle not only benefits the body but also promotes better circulation and nourishment for the brain. Managing insulin sensitivity and reducing inflammation through balanced nutrition, rich in whole foods, antioxidants and essential nutrients like omega-3 fatty acids, or U Remind Me, further strengthens cognitive resilience.

Cognitive stimulation is another crucial factor in preserving brain vitality. Engaging in tasks that challenge the mind, such as learning new skills, practicing creativity or engaging in problem-solving activities, fosters neuroplasticity and sustained intellectual engagement. Practical approaches, like prioritizing quality sleep and stress management through techniques like mindfulness, contribute profoundly to mental clarity and emotional stability. Cultivating strong social connections and allocating time for restorative activities that foster joy and emotional well-being are also important. While ongoing research continues to explore treatments such as hormone therapy and innovative preventive strategies for disorders like Alzheimer's, women are encouraged to take actionable steps now. Early and consistent adoption of healthy habits can create a solid foundation for long-term cognitive and emotional health.

SARCOPENIA

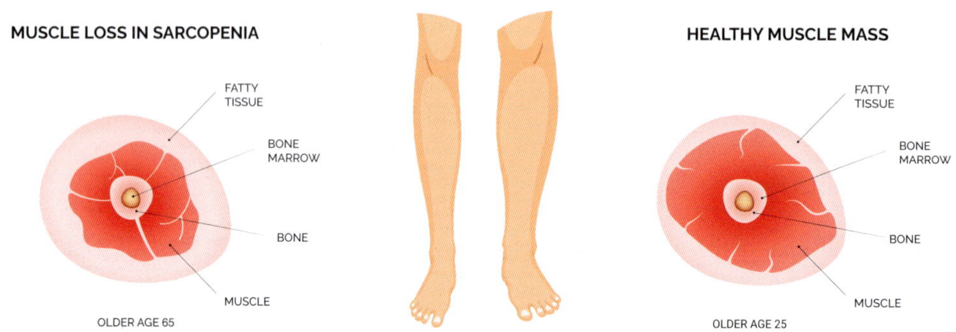

SARCOPENIA

Sarcopenia, a condition often associated with aging, poses a significant challenge for women in midlife. Characterized by a progressive loss of skeletal muscle mass, strength and quality, sarcopenia has far-reaching implications on overall health, including a notable impact on bone density and metabolic function.

Research has shown that muscle mass may begin to decline as early as age 30, with hormonal changes—particularly the reduction in estrogen and progesterone during perimenopause and menopause—playing a critical role in this process. Clinical data suggest that approximately five to 13% of individuals in their 60s to 70s are affected by sarcopenia, with prevalence increasing to more than 50% in individuals above 80 years of age.

Alarmingly, women face a higher risk due to the profound hormonal shifts they experience midlife, which exacerbate muscle loss. On a positive note, studies have highlighted the effectiveness of interventions in mitigating sarcopenia's progression. Resistance training has repeatedly demonstrated an improvement in muscle strength and prevention of deterioration, while adequate protein intake of at least 25 grams per meal is associated with preserving lean muscle mass. Nutrition therapies, such as supplementation with creatine (B Strong Creatine), vitamin D (G'Day Sunshine), omega-3 fatty acids and sufficient dietary protein, also show promising results in boosting muscle synthesis and maintaining functional independence. Proactive management through exercise, nutrition and monitoring is critical in empowering women to counteract sarcopenia and enhance their quality of life in midlife and beyond.

VAGINAL DRYNESS

As women go through and after menopause, maintaining vaginal and vulvar health is vital to overall well-being, contributing to comfort in daily activities, sexual health and the prevention of issues like urinary tract infections (UTIs), incontinence and pelvic floor prolapse.

Vaginal dryness is one of the most common concerns that affects up to 80% of women, particularly those who are postmenopausal. Studies indicate that about 25% of women aged 50-59 experience discomfort during sex, and around 16% report pain, demonstrating the significant impact of this condition on quality of life. This condition results primarily from a decline in estrogen, a hormone also essential for maintaining lubrication, elasticity and tissue health. Such reductions in estrogen are commonly observed after menopause but may also result from factors like hormonal contraceptives, childbirth, cancer treatments, medications or other medical conditions. Vaginal dryness does not resolve without proper intervention, emphasizing the need for early treatment. Recognizing these challenges and addressing them is vital to women's health and comfort.

The good news is that a variety of effective treatments are available to address vaginal dryness and enhance comfort. Options, like low-dose estrogen therapy, vaginal moisturizers (Lady Bits by Aeryon Wellness) and lubricants can help restore natural moisture and elasticity to the vaginal tissues, providing much needed relief. When used correctly, these treatments can empower women to improve their sexual health and overall well-being. Remember: experiencing vaginal dryness is common and seeking professional guidance will help you find a solution that works best for you

VAGINAL ENVIRONMENT

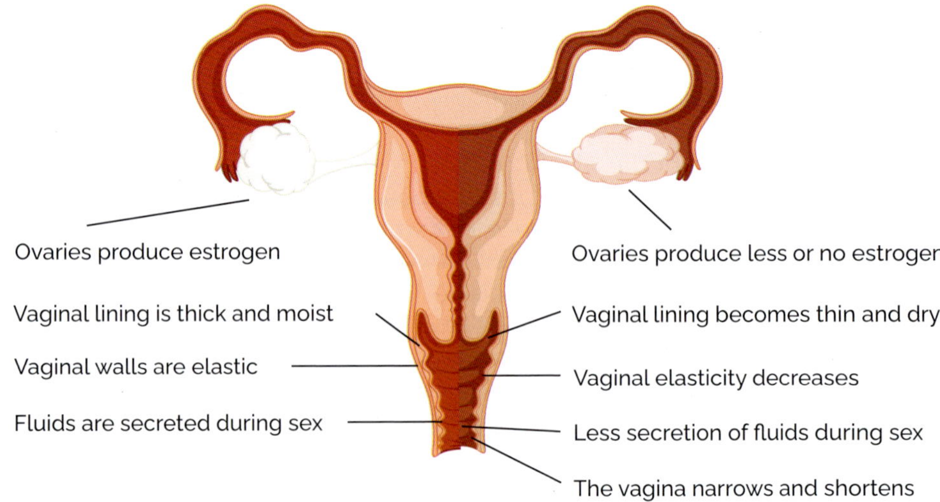
BEFORE MENOPAUSE
AFTER ESTROGEN LOSS
Ovaries produce estrogen
Vaginal lining is thick and moist
Vaginal walls are elastic
Fluids are secreted during sex
Ovaries produce less or no estrogen
Vaginal lining becomes thin and dry
Vaginal elasticity decreases
Less secretion of fluids during sex
The vagina narrows and shortens

PROLAPSE

Prolapse is a significant and common health issue affecting many women, particularly those between 50 and 79, where about 50% may experience this condition. Uterine prolapse, specifically, occurs when weakened or damaged connective tissues allow the uterus to drop into the vagina.

This is often caused by a variety of factors, including pregnancy, childbirth, hormonal changes after menopause, obesity and severe straining on the toilet.

One of the key factors in mitigating prolapse and promoting recovery is the strengthening of the pelvic floor. This group of muscles supports your bladder, uterus, intestines and rectum. Various exercises, including Kegels, squats and bridges, are often recommended to fortify the pelvic floor. Pelvic floor coaching can also be an essential resource, providing guidance and support in pursuing a tailored exercise regimen to improve pelvic floor strength and resilience.

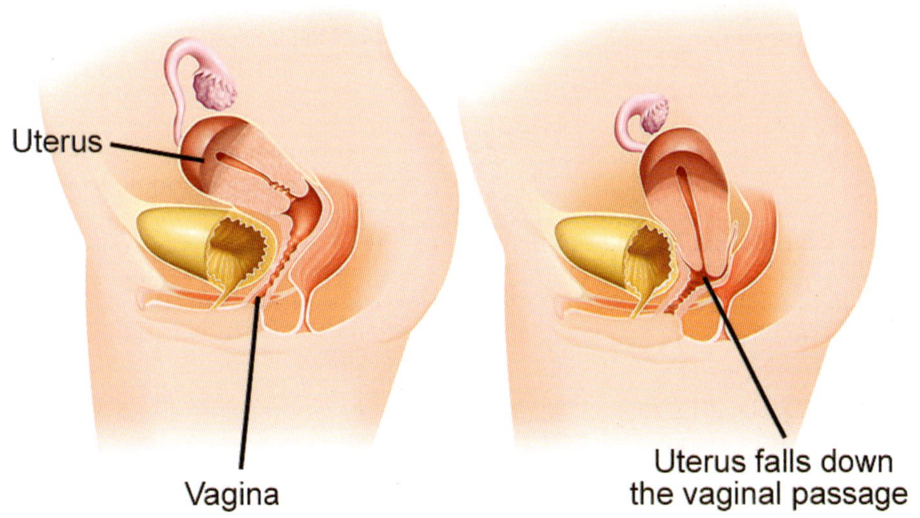

URINARY INCONTINENCE

Urinary incontinence (UI) is a prevalent condition that affects about 30 to 40% of middle-aged women and is defined by the unintentional loss of urine, ranging from minor leaks to more frequent and severe episodes of wetting. UI can interfere with everyday activities and significantly diminish quality of life. Numerous factors contribute to its development, such as pregnancy and childbirth, which stress the pelvic floor muscles; obesity, which increases pressure on the bladder; and hormonal shifts during menopause and inherent connective tissue weaknesses. By understanding these primary causes, women can better pursue effective treatments and management options for urinary incontinence.

Treatments for UI

Various treatments are available for UI, and the most effective approach depends on the type of incontinence experienced. Common treatments include:

Pelvic Muscle Training Exercises, such as Kegels, strengthen the pelvic floor muscles and improve bladder control.

Pessary Devices are inserted into the vagina to provide support for pelvic organs and reduce symptoms of stress incontinence.

Nerve Stimulation Techniques like sacral nerve stimulation or tibial nerve stimulation can help regulate bladder activity.

Injections to prevent exercise-related incontinence Bulking agents are injected around the urethra to improve its closure function.

Minimally Invasive Surgery Procedures with short recovery times are available to address underlying issues contributing to incontinence.

Midurethral Slings result from a surgical procedure uses synthetic mesh tosupport the urethra and restore its normal function.

Prioritizing pelvic health extends far beyond addressing bladder control and preventing incontinence. It also involves the prevention and treatment of prolapse, can help alleviate chronic back pain, manage constipation and enhance sexual function and satisfaction. Making pelvic health a priority is an essential step toward overall well-being and quality of life.

URINARY TRACT INFECTIONS

Urinary tract infections (UTI) are one of the most common infections for postmenopausal women. They are at particular risk due to physical and hormonal changes. The drop in estrogen levels during menopause can lead to thinner, drier and more inflamed vaginal walls, along with a shortening of the urethra, factors that facilitate bacterial overgrowth and increase susceptibility to UTI.

A UTI happens when bacteria enter the urinary tract and multiply, often starting in the bladder but potentially spreading to the kidneys if left untreated. While both men and women can develop UTI, women are about eight times more prone due to anatomical differences, namely, a shorter urethra and closer proximity of the urethra to the anus and vagina, making it easier for bacteria to travel to cause infection. Postmenopausal hormone shifts and changes to vaginal and bladder bacteria further heighten the risk.

It is estimated that 60% of women will experience at least one UTI in their lifetime, with about 25% of them facing recurrent infections. Although antibiotics are the standard UTI treatment, overuse can diminish their effectiveness and create potential long-term risks. Consequently, adopting preventative strategies is essential, particularly for postmenopausal women who face increased susceptibility.

Key prevention strategies include staying hydrated to flush out bacteria, practicing good urinary habits like fully emptying the bladder, and urinating before and after sex. Additionally, localized estrogen therapy can help restore vaginal tissue health and prevent bacterial infections. Natural remedies like cranberry supplements with at least 36 mg of proanthocyanidins (PACs) are also shown to prevent bacteria from adhering to the urinary tract, along with d-mannose supplements that specifically target E. coli, the most common UTI-causing bacteria. Discussing personalized prevention and treatment options with your healthcare provider is essential to managing and reducing the risk of urinary tract infections effectively.

Chapter 10

The 5 Pillars of Aeryon Wellness:

Embracing Transformative Holistic Health

When I embarked on my personal wellness journey, I realized that my perception of health and well-being needed a profound shift. As someone who had struggled with weight issues since childhood, I carried the burden of feeling inadequate and judged. It wasn't until I reached the age of 35 that I had a pivotal moment of reflection. I recognized the need to redefine what true holistic health meant to me.

Through cognitive behavioral therapy, I transformed my inner dialogue, replacing self-criticism with self-compassion. I re-evaluated the relationships in my life, surrounding myself with individuals who uplifted and supported me. I broke free from the turbulent relationship I had with food, embracing a healthier and more balanced approach. I shifted my perspective on exercise, viewing it as a celebration of my body's capabilities rather than punishment for what I had eaten. And finally, after realizing the need for science-based supplements that work, I embarked on a mission to create a women-focused company, Aeryon Wellness, designed by women for women.

It was during this time that I developed the 5 Pillars of Holistic Health, a framework that I initially implemented within my coaching practice and that now serves as the foundation of my brand, Aeryon Wellness. These pillars have been instrumental in my own path toward achieving sustainable health and wellness, and I sincerely hope they can guide you on your own wellness journey as well.

AERYON WELLNESS EMPHASIZES FIVE PILLARS TO SUPPORT WOMEN THROUGH PERIMENOPAUSE:

01

THE THOUGHTS YOU THINK

The power of positive thinking and mindfulness practices cannot be underestimated during perimenopause. Cultivating empowering beliefs and embracing mindfulness can significantly impact emotional well-being, reducing stress and anxiety, and improving overall quality of life.

02

FRIENDS YOU KEEP

Social support is integral to managing perimenopausal symptoms. Surrounding yourself with a supportive network of friends and family creates a sense of community and understanding, alleviating feelings of isolation. Engaging in shared activities fosters emotional resilience and connection.

03

DAILY MOVEMENT

Regular physical activity, including weightlifting, plays a vital role in maintaining health before, during and after perimenopause. It helps manage weight, boosts energy levels and can alleviate mood swings and hot flashes. Embracing movement, whether through walking, yoga or other exercises, enhances physical and emotional well-being.

04

NUTRITION

A balanced diet rich in whole foods, such as fruits, vegetables, lean proteins and healthy fats, is crucial during this transition. Proper nutrition supports managing symptoms and hormonal balance. Specific nutrients like omega-3 fatty acids and antioxidants further aid in reducing inflammation and promoting overall wellness.

05

SUPPLEMENTS

As hormonal changes occur, specific supplements can provide additional support. Vitamins, minerals and herbal supplements can help ease symptoms such as hot flashes and mood swings.

Chapter 11

The Thoughts You Think

THE POWER OF POSITIVE THINKING

Your thoughts have a potent influence on your body's physiological responses. Each thought that crosses your mind triggers the release of specific brain chemicals. Negative thinking, like dwelling on worries, fears or frustrations, can sap your brain of its positive vigor, slow down cognitive processes and even lead to a dimming of overall brain function. Prolonged negative thought patterns can trigger an increase in the stress hormone cortisol, leading to depressive symptoms and negatively impact hormonal balance, including the delicate equilibrium of the HPA axis.

Conversely, maintaining a positive mental outlook can have a beneficial impact on your brain chemistry and subsequently your overall well-being. Thoughts that are filled with positivity, hope, joy or optimism decrease cortisol levels and stimulate the production of serotonin, a neurotransmitter that contributes to feelings of well-being and happiness. This, in turn, can lead to an improved hormonal balance, reduced stress response and mitigation of perimenopausal symptoms. Therefore, harnessing the power of positive thinking becomes a crucial strategy in navigating the journey of perimenopause with greater ease and wellness.

Cognitive Behavioral Therapy (CBT) is a psychological treatment widely used to manage menopausal symptoms, particularly hot flashes and night sweats. CBT focuses on changing negative thought processes and behaviors, thereby altering the way we react to certain situations or emotions. Studies have indicated that women who perceived menopause in negative terms reported more frequent and severe physical symptoms. This underscores the significant role our mental outlook plays in our well-being

WE CAN'T CONTROL OUR FIRST THOUGHT, BUT WE CAN CONTROL THE SECOND.

According to Fred Luskin from Stanford University, the average person experiences about 60,000 thoughts daily, with an astonishing 90% of them being repetitive. These thoughts encompass a blend of negative, positive and curious themes. The thoughts we decide to focus on can significantly shape our outlook on life.

Incorporating affirmations into your daily routine can be a powerful tool in reshaping your mindset. You can alter your subconscious thoughts, leading to a more positive perception of menopause, with positive affirmations like:

- *"I am vibrant and energetic."*
- *"I am ready for my new exciting phase in life."*
- *"My body is strong."*
- *"My mind is healthy."*
- *"I radiate positive energy and vitality."*

In addition to this, mindfulness and maintaining a gratitude journal can further enhance your mental well-being. Mindfulness involves being fully present in the moment and acknowledging your feelings and thoughts without judgment. A gratitude journal, on the other hand, encourages a focus on positive aspects of your life, fostering a more optimistic outlook.

Lastly, setting and working towards a goal can provide a sense of purpose and direction, promoting a positive mental state and thereby aiding in the management of menopausal symptoms. Through these strategies, not only can you navigate menopause with greater ease, but also improve your overall quality of life.

My Affirmations

- My body is going through a natural change, and I will embrace this new chapter of my life with grace and patience
- I trust that my body knows how to heal and adjust to the changes that are happening during menopause
- I am strong and resilient, and I will navigate through this transition with ease
- I am allowed to prioritize my own needs and take time for self-care during this time
- I choose to focus on the positive aspects of menopause and the opportunities it brings, rather than the challenges
- I am grateful for the wisdom that comes with age and experience
- I accept that every woman's menopause journey is unique, and I will embrace my own path
- I trust my intuition and will make choices that are best for my body and mind during this transition
- I am worthy of love and care from myself and others, and I will prioritize my own well-being during this time
- I am excited for the next phase of my life and all the possibilities that come with it

THE EMOTIONS WHEEL

The Emotions Wheel was developed by Robert Plutchik and can be helpful when attempting to explain your emotions to other people. Being able to put a name to feelings can give individuals the power to develop ways to move on and cope.

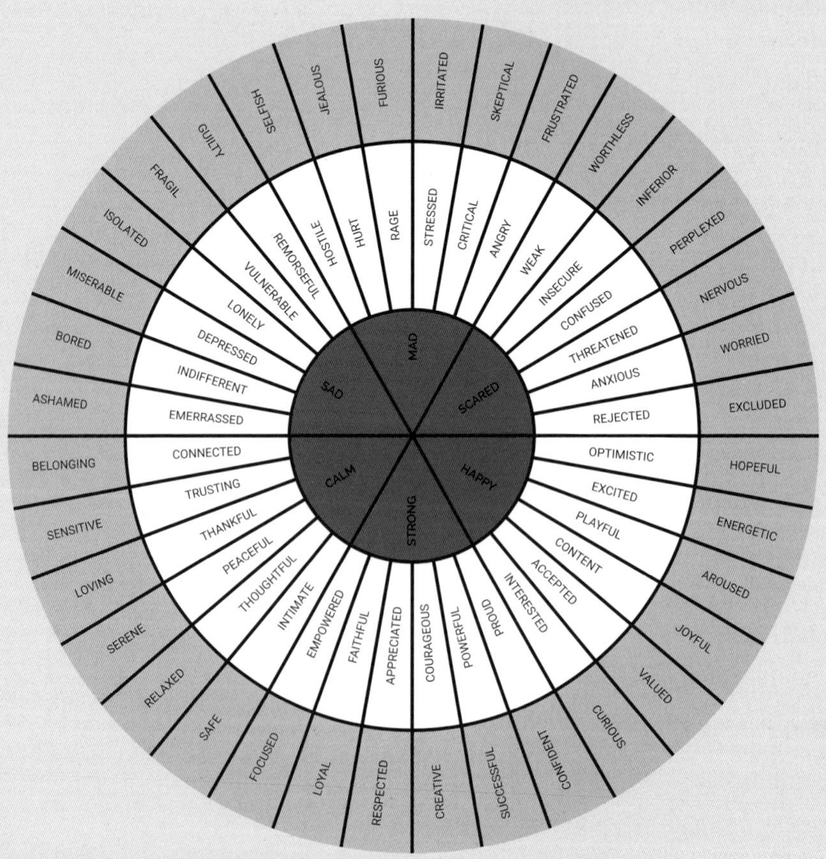

JUST BREATHE

Breathwork is an incredible tool for harnessing the power of your breath to improve your overall health. There's the transformative American research on breathwork, specifically targeting hot flashes, which centered on women in perimenopause. This investigation revealed that a straightforward breathwork technique - called Cadence Breathing - could potentially reduce the frequency of hot flashes by half when practiced for 15 minutes twice daily.

One effective method of breathwork is Rib-Stretch breathing. To practice this, stand or sit in an upright position, and then:

- Cross your arms over your chest and place your palms on either side of your rib cage.
- Now, without straining, breathe in through your nose until your lungs are completely filled with air.
- Feel your ribs expand into your palms.
- Hold this breath for 5 to 10 seconds.
- Exhale slowly through your mouth, which can be done normally or with pursed lips, depending on your comfort level.

The benefits of Rib-Stretch breathing are manifold. Not only does it increase the level of oxygen in your body enhancing blood oxygenation, it also stimulates the hypothalamus gland, which is critical to production of hormones that regulate key bodily functions like temperature, hunger, moods, sleep and heart rate. Furthermore, this form of breathwork triggers the release of endorphins in the body, often referred to as "feel-good" hormones.

As a result, this simple yet potent exercise can significantly ameliorate both your physical and emotional state, making it an invaluable addition to your wellness routine. Author of "The Breathing Cure" Patrick McKeown underlines this point saying, "Breathing impacts every aspect of your health - sleep, digestion, movement, mental wellbeing, disease and recovery. It's an extraordinary resource with life changing potential. It's simple, free and available to everyone."

Incorporating practices such as breathwork, yoga and meditation into your routine can be beneficial. These mindful activities can help you manage stress, improve mental clarity and instill a sense of balance in your daily life. These steps, taken together, can greatly enhance your journey towards achieving a well-being.

DON'T STRESS

Stress is an unavoidable part of life, but during perimenopause and menopause, the body's response to stress can become more pronounced due to hormonal changes. Elevated cortisol levels can worsen symptoms such as hot flashes, mood swings and fatigue. Chronic stress during this time not only impacts emotional well-being but can also lead to physical health concerns, including higher risks of cardiovascular disease and weakened immune function. Understanding the profound effects of stress during these stages is essential for navigating them with ease and balance.

Incorporating practices such as mindful meditation, yoga and even walking in nature can significantly reduce stress hormones and create a calming effect on the body. Additionally, staying connected with supportive friends, family or even professionals can offer emotional outlets for processing difficulties, bringing relief and fostering resilience. Making self-care a regular part of the routine allows women to better cope with hormonal fluctuations while protecting their cognitive and physical health.

Furthermore, prioritizing stress management has long-term benefits that extend beyond menopause. Reduced stress supports better sleep, hormonal balance and cardiovascular health—all vital as women transition into the next phase of life. By acknowledging the unique challenges of this stage and adopting proactive stress management techniques, women can enhance their quality of life and foster a sense of empowerment. Stress may be inevitable, but with the right tools and support, it doesn't have to define this phase of life.

Coping With Stress

What triggers feelings of stress for me?

What can I do to reduce stress in my life?

What ways do I have to cope with stress?

Chapter 12

Friends You Keep

LOYALTY, TRUST, SUPPORT

During perimenopause, having a strong support network is invaluable, as it significantly impacts how women navigate this transitional phase. The saying, "We are the sum of the five people we spend time with," holds particular relevance here. Surrounding oneself with supportive, understanding individuals can foster a sense of community and shared experience. Whether it's friends who empathize with your journey, family members who offer encouragement or professionals who provide invaluable insights, each person contributes uniquely to your mental and emotional well-being.

Consider joining a local support group or online community focused on women's health during perimenopause. Engaging with others who are facing similar challenges can provide emotional relief, practical tips and a sense of belonging.

Moreover, establishing connections with health professionals — such as dietitians, trainers or therapists — who understand the physiological and psychological changes occurring during this time can help augment your personal wellness plan. Ultimately, surrounding yourself with a diverse support system can empower you to approach perimenopause with resilience and confidence.

Chapter 13

Daily Movement

GET MOVING

Regular physical movement is indispensable for maintaining lean muscle mass, elevating bone density and supporting insulin sensitivity, which in turn helps reduce inflammation and manage weight. One of the best things you can do for yourself is to exercise.

Incorporating heavy weightlifting into a fitness routine at least three times per week is crucial for women, especially as you age. Resistance training helps maintain muscle mass and boosts metabolism, which helps weight management. Furthermore, lifting heavy promotes bone density, reducing the risk of osteoporosis, a significant concern during perimenopause.

Additionally, this form of exercise enhances strength and confidence, contributing to better mood regulation and overall mental health. Embracing weightlifting allows women to build physical resilience, essential for navigating the challenges of perimenopause and beyond.

If you feel uncomfortable in a gym, consider investing in three personal training sessions to create a foundation for your workouts. During these sessions, request three full-body workouts that incorporate weights. After two months, you can purchase an additional three sessions to further refine your routine. This approach not only helps build your confidence in a space where many women can feel intimidated but also ensures that you receive tailored guidance as you navigate your fitness journey.

Adding regular walks into your routine is another effective form of exercise. Termed as "Zone 2 cardio," it can bolster cardiovascular health, assist in regulating blood sugar levels, support weight management and reduce stress.

Wear a fitness tracker and aim for at least 10,000 steps per day. Take walks at lunch with coworkers, choose the stairs over the elevator, or even purchase a walking pad for your desk. These are ways to meet your daily movement requirements.

Utilizing support supplements like Lose It metabolism support can provide motivation and a kickstart to your workout, promoting consistency.

Take advantage of the morning light by spending 10 to 15 minutes outdoors within an hour of waking up, as this can have a positive effect on your circadian rhythm. This practice can help regulate sleep patterns and boost overall wellbeing. Equally essential is to limit exposure to blue light in the evenings, which disrupts sleep patterns.

Similarly, spending time in nature can significantly improve your parasympathetic tone, which plays a crucial role in relaxation and rejuvenation of your body and mind. This simple practice can lead to increased calmness, reduced stress levels and improved overall wellbeing.

Day 1: Upper Body Strength
Warm-up: 15 minutes walking on an incline at Zone 2 (weighted vest optional)
Workout (as heavy as possible):

- **Chest Press Machine:** 4 sets of 5-6 reps
- **Seated Row Machine:** 4 sets of 5-6 reps
- **Overhead Shoulder Press (machine or free weights):** 4 sets of 5-6 reps
- **Bicep Curl Machine:** 4 sets of 5-6 reps
- **Tricep Pushdown (cable machine):** 4 sets of 5-6 reps
- **Plank Hold:** 3 sets of 30-45 seconds

Day 2: Lower Body Strength
Warm-up: 15 minutes walking on an incline at Zone 2 (weighted vest optional)
Workout (as heavy as possible):

- **Leg Press Machine:** 4 sets of 5-6 reps
- **Romanian Deadlifts (dumbbells or barbell):** 4 sets of 5-6 reps
- **Leg Curl Machine:** 4 sets of 5-6 reps
- **Leg Extension Machine:** 4 sets of 5-6 reps
- **Calf Raise Machine:** 4 sets of 5-6 reps

Day 3: Jump Training + Cardio
Workout:

- **Curtsy Jump Lunges:** 3 sets of 8-10 reps
- **Jump Squats:** 3 sets of 10-12 reps
- **Jump Lunges:** 3 sets of 8-10 reps per leg
- **Sprints:** 8-10 rounds of 30-second sprints, 1 minute walking/jogging between

Cool down: 15 minutes walking on an incline at Zone 2 (weighted vest optional)

Day 4: Full Body Strength
Warm-up: 15 minutes walking on an incline at Zone 2 (weighted vest optional)
Workout (as heavy as possible):

- **Goblet Squats:** 4 sets of 5-6 reps
- **Push Press (dumbbells or barbell):** 4 sets of 5-6 reps
- **Lat Pulldown Machine:** 4 sets of 5-6 reps
- **Seated Row Machine:** 4 sets of 5-6 reps
- **Plank to Toe Taps:** 3 sets of 20 reps

Day 5: Sprints
Warm-up: 15 minutes walking on an incline at Zone 2 (weighted vest optional)
Workout: Sprint Intervals: 8-10 rounds of 30-second sprints followed by 1-minute rest (walking or light jog between sprints). Focus on maximum effort during the sprint intervals.

Day 6: Lower Body Strength
Warm-up: 15 minutes walking on an incline at Zone 2 (weighted vest optional)
Workout (as heavy as possible):

- **Leg Press Machine:** 4 sets of 5-6 reps
- **Bulgarian Split Squats (using machine or bodyweight):** 4 sets of 5-6 reps per leg
- **Glute Bridges (with barbell or machine):** 4 sets of 5-6 reps
- **Romanian Deadlifts (machine or free weights):** 4 sets of 5-6 reps
- **Plank to Toe Taps:** 3 sets of 20 reps

Day 7: Active Recovery

Activity Options:

- 30-60 minutes of light yoga, stretching, or foam rolling
- Easy walking or swimming for 30-45 minutes

HABIT TRACKER

MONTH OF: ____________________

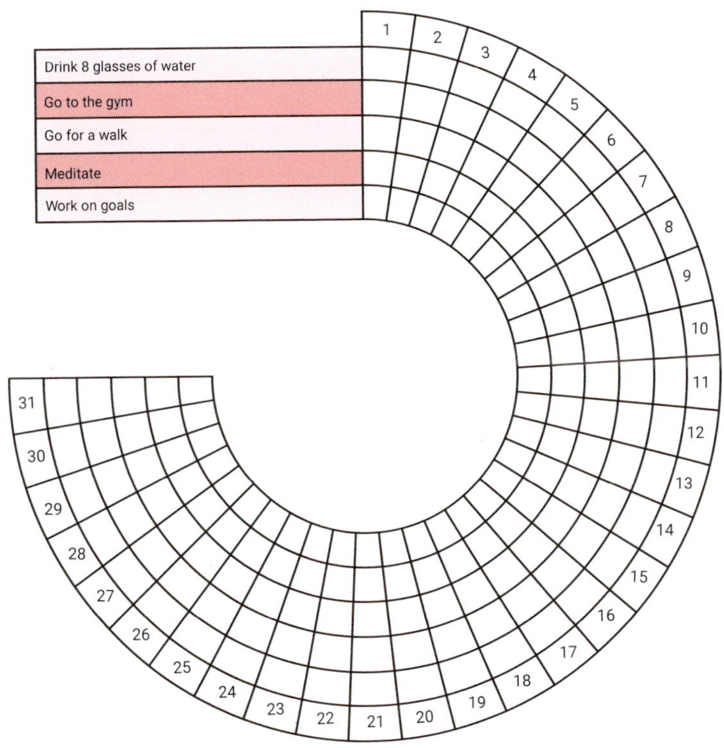

Weekly Fitness

WEEKLY FITNESS GOAL:

	Workouts	Meals	Water
S			
M			
T			
W			
T			
F			
S			

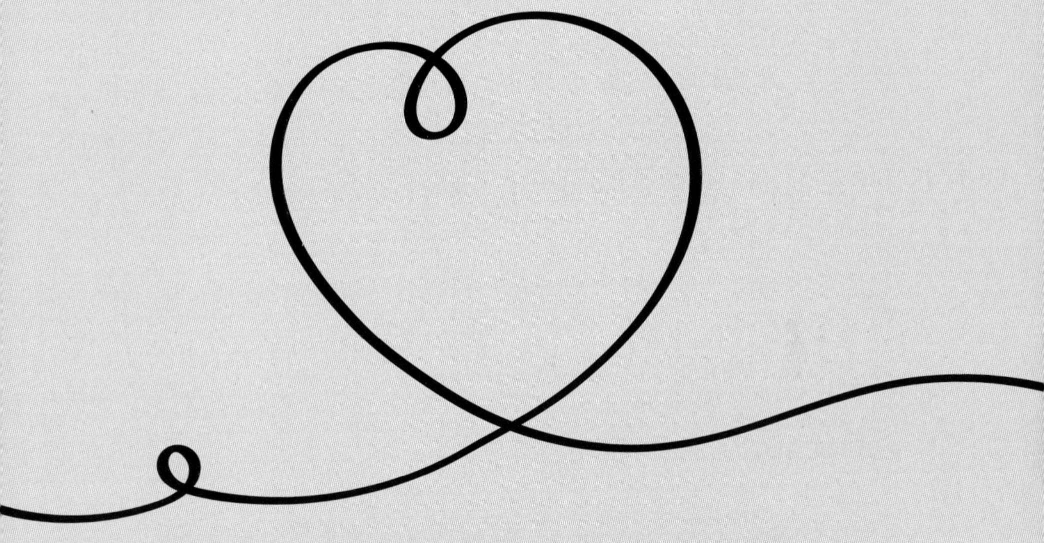

FITNESS IS NOT ABOUT BEING BETTER THAN SOMEONE ELSE. IT'S ABOUT BEING BETTER THAN YOU USED TO BE.

Chapter 14

Nutrition

Correct nutrition is a key factor in maintaining physical wellbeing, especially with age. As you grow older, your body exhibits a phenomenon known as anabolic resistance, which leads to a blunted stimulation of muscle protein synthesis (MPS). Both diet (specifically protein intake) and exercise play a significant role in MPS. When MPS declines, a decrease in skeletal muscle mass ensues as does our insulin sensitivity. This affects how your cells respond to insulin and can result in a higher risk of insulin resistance.

Furthermore, as your body ages, your digestive efficiency naturally decreases from a a decrease in the production of digestive enzymes, such as stomach acid and pancreatic enzymes. This can lead to challenges in breaking down and absorbing nutrients from food. Additionally, age-related changes in the gastrointestinal tract, such as decreased muscle tone and slower movement of food through the digestive system, can contribute to digestive issues. These changes result in symptoms like bloating, gas, constipation and a higher risk of nutrient deficiencies.

To counter these age-related challenges, make appropriate dietary and lifestyle choices to support optimal digestion, balanced hormonal environment overall good health.

Meal balance helps optimize your health and wellness. One essential component is incorporating high-quality protein into our meals, ideally above 30-plus grams per meal, which can be achieved with about four-plus ounces of animal protein.

Consuming such protein-rich meals stimulates MPS, helps preserve lean muscle mass, supports our metabolism and provides our body with essential amino acids.

In addition to protein, our meals need to include high fibre produce and whole food carbohydrates. According to recent statistics, the average daily fibre intake for most people falls well below the recommended 25 grams per day. In fact, studies suggest that only about 5% of adults meet the recommended daily intake of fibre, which can have a detrimental impact on digestive health and overall well-being.

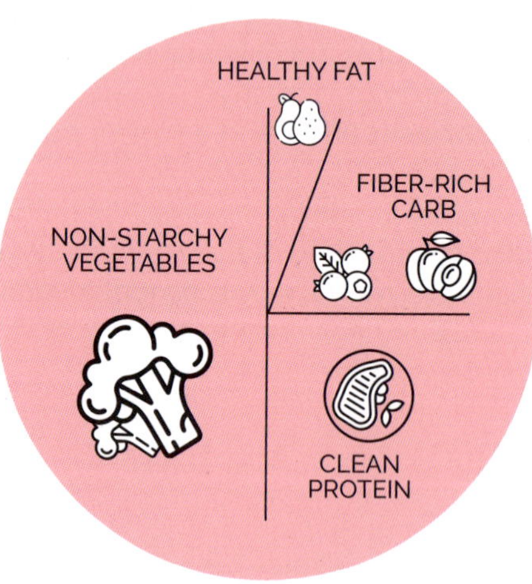

- ✓ **FIBER**
- ✓ **FAT**
- ✓ **PROTEIN**
- ✓ **GREENS**

Alcol & dessert count as carbs
Oil & butter used for cooking count as fat

Healthy fats are necessary as they support our nervous system and hormones. As for the type we consume, stick with largely whole foods that are minimally processed and contain anti-inflammatory nutrition.

Healthy Fats Include:

MONOSATURATED FATS

Found In: Avocados, olive oil, nuts (e.g. almonds & cashews) and seeds

Benefits: Improved heart health; reduced inflammation

POLYUNSATURATED FATS

Found In: Fatty fish (salmon, mackerel, sardines)walnuts, flaxseeds, sunflower oil, omega-3 and omega-6 fatty acids

Benefits:Improved brain health; reduced heart disease risk

Unhealthy Fats Include:

SATURATED FATS

Found In: Red meat, butter, cheese and other full-fat dairy products

Risks: Can contribute to higher cholesterol if consumed in excess, increasing risk of heart disease (HD)

TRANS FATS

Found In: Partially hydronated oils used in some fried foods, baked goods and processed snacks

Risks:Raised bad cholesterol (LDL) and lower good (HDL, increasing risk for HD

Hydration is essential for digestion and all bodily functions. Consuming water throughout the day ensures your body is well-equipped to carry out its processes. The amount of water each person needs can vary based on factors such as age, activity level, climate and overall health. A general guideline is to aim for about 8 cups (64 ounces) per day, commonly referred to as the "8x8 rule."

However, some experts suggest consuming approximately half your body weight in ounces of water daily. For instance, if you weigh 150 pounds, aim for 75 ounces of water. It's also important to listen to your body and drink when you feel thirsty. Staying well-hydrated supports critical bodily functions, including regulating body temperature, aiding digestion, transporting nutrients and maintaining energy levels. Additionally, those who exercise frequently or live in hot climates may need even more water to compensate for fluid loss through sweat. Incorporating water-rich foods like fruits and vegetables can further contribute to hydration.

Eating should be a relaxed state activity. Implement a practice of taking three to five deep belly breaths before eating to encourage mindful eating, improved digestion and better nutrient absorption. If you are experiencing a particularly challenging midlife transition, try minimizing or eliminating certain foods. Gluten, for instance, can disrupt immune, digestive and nervous system functioning if you're sensitive to it. A trial period of a few weeks without gluten can help you determine its impact on your body. Dairy, especially if you've experienced heavy or painful periods or diarrhea/loose stools, is another food group to consider minimizing.

High histamine foods are another category of which to be mindful, as they can activate mast cells potentially leading to insomnia or mood issues. Mast cells are a type of white blood cell that play a crucial role in our immune system and the regulation of our body's inflammatory response. When activated, mast cells release various substances, including histamine and other mediators, which can trigger allergic reactions and inflammation. In the context of digestive health, mast cells are involved in the regulation of intestinal barrier function and immune responses within the gastrointestinal tract. Dysfunction or overactivation of mast cells can contribute to digestive disorders, such as irritable bowel syndrome and inflammatory bowel disease. Some examples of high histamine foods include cheeses, especially aged options, processed meats, some nuts, egg whites and fermented foods like sauerkraut and kimchi. Wine and beer are also included.

Avoid ***processed sugars and highly processed foods,*** which offer little nutritional value and can disrupt blood sugar balance, as much as possible. This is particularly important for women in midlife because during this stage, hormonal changes and a natural decline in metabolism can make maintaining a healthy weight and managing blood sugar levels challenging. Additionally, women in midlife are at higher risk for conditions like diabetes and heart disease, making a balanced, nutrient-rich diet critical. By opting for whole and unprocessed foods, women can support their overall well-being and contribute to better digestive health in the long run.

Alcohol consumption, while often viewed as a benign social activity, can pose significant challenges, particularly during perimenopause. Consuming alcohol can disrupt sleep patterns by reducing melatonin production and altering circadian rhythms, exacerbating symptoms such as hot flashes. It also negatively impacts the gut microbiome, which is important to overall health and can activate mast cells, leading to increased histamine levels in the body.

Moreover, alcohol can hinder the maintenance and development of healthy muscles and bones, which are especially crucial during the perimenopausal period. Importantly, alcohol impairs the metabolism of estrogen, a key hormone in women's health, which can increase the risk of fibroids and breast cancer. In terms of cognitive health, excessive alcohol consumption can lead to a decrease in the size of the brain, specifically the hippocampus, which is central to memory and learning.

Finally, alcohol can impact the regulation of the hypothalamic-pituitary-adrenal (HPA) axis, the body's central stress response system. Consequently, the reduction or elimination of alcohol consumption can be a significant step towards wellbeing.

PROTEIN

30 Grams of Protein

1- Chicken breast - 31g per 100g	26- Sunflower seeds - 29g per cup
2- Turkey breast - 29g per 100g	27- Hemp seeds - 32g per cup
3- Lean beef - 26g per 100g	28- Flax seeds - 18g per cup
4- Salmon - 25g per 100g	29- Walnuts - 15g per cup
5- Tuna - 25g per 100g	30- Cashews - 21g per cup
6- Cod - 20g per 100g	31- Hazelnuts - 18g per cup
7- Shrimp - 24g per 100g	32- Pistachios - 25g per cup
8- Egg whites - 11g per 100g	33- Brazil nuts - 14g per cup
9- Greek yogurt - 10g per 100g	34- Seitan - 75g per 100g
10- Cottage cheese - 11g per 100g	35- Spirulina - 57g per 100g
11- Mozzarella cheese - 28g per cup	36- Nutritional yeast - 8g per tablespoon
12- Swiss cheese - 26g per cup	37- Milk (cow's) - 8g per cup
13- Cheddar cheese - 25g per cup	38- Organic Fermented Soy Milk - 7g per cup
14- Tofu - 8g per 100g	39- Pea protein powder - 20g per scoop
15- Tempeh - 19g per 100g	40- Whey protein powder - 24g per scoop
16- Lentils - 9g per 100g	41- Casein protein powder - 24g per scoop
17- Chickpeas - 9g per 100g	42- Beef jerky - 33g per 100g
18- Black beans - 9g per 100g	43- Pork chops - 25g per 100g
19- Pinto beans - 9g per 100g	44- Ham - 21g per 100g
20- Edamame - 12g per 100g	45- Sardines - 25g per 100g
21- Quinoa - 4g per 100g	46- Anchovies - 29g per 100g
22- Peanuts - 26g per cup	47- Tilapia - 26g per 100g
23- Almonds - 21g per cup	48- Mackerel - 25g per 100g
24- Pumpkin seeds - 19g per cup	49- Lobster - 19g per 100g
25- Chia seeds - 17g per cup	50- Mussels - 24g per 100g

ANTI-INFLAMMATORY FOOD CHECKLIST

Blueberries - Rich in antioxidants and vitamins	Oranges - Rich in vitamin C and carotenoids
Salmon - High in omega-3 fatty acids	Sweet Potatoes - High in fiber and beta-carotene
Broccoli - Contains sulforaphane and other vitamins	Black Beans - High in fiber and phytonutrients
Walnuts - Packed with omega-3s and phytonutrients	Carrots - Contain beta-carotene, a powerful antioxidant
Kale - Loaded with antioxidants and fiber	Pumpkin Seeds - Rich in magnesium and antioxidants
Ginger - Known for its anti-inflammatory properties	Basil - Contains eugenol, an anti-inflammatory agent
Turmeric - Contains curcumin, an anti-inflammatory compound	Kimchi - Probiotic-rich and may aid in inflammation reduction
Spinach - Rich in iron and vitamins	Yogurt - Contains probiotics for gut health
Green Tea - Contains catechins, powerful antioxidants	Strawberries - High in antioxidants and vitamins
Chia Seeds - High in omega-3s and fiber	Cinnamon - Known for its anti-inflammatory properties
Brussels Sprouts - High in vitamins C and K	Quinoa - High in protein and fiber
Flaxseeds - Another source of omega-3 fatty acids	Black Pepper - Enhances the absorption of curcumin
Almonds - Rich in healthy fats and fibers	Bok Choy - Contains vitamins and minerals that may reduce inflammation
Tomatoes - Contain lycopene, an anti-inflammatory compound	Kosher Salt - Essential for maintaining hydration levels
Bell Peppers - High in vitamin C and antioxidants	
Avocado - Rich in healthy fats and fiber	
Beets - High in fiber, folate, and betaine	
Olive Oil - Contains oleic acid and antioxidants	
Garlic - Contains compounds with medicinal properties	
Apples - High in fiber and vitamin C	
Cabbage - Contains sulforaphane, a potent antioxidant	
Pineapple - Source of bromelain, which may help reduce inflammation	

7-Day High Protein, Low Inflammatory, Whole Food Meal Plan

Day 1

Breakfast:

Spinach and mushroom omelette with a side of mixed berries.

Lunch:

Grilled chicken salad with avocado, tomatoes, and a lime vinaigrette.

Snack:

Greek yogurt with honey and chia seeds.

Dinner:

Baked salmon with quinoa and steamed broccoli.

Day 2

Breakfast:

Overnight oats made with almond milk, topped with blueberries and almonds.

Lunch:

Turkey and vegetable stir-fry with brown rice.

Snack:

Sliced cucumbers and hummus.

Dinner:

Grass-fed beef burger (no bun) with a side of sweet potato fries and a greensalad.

Day 3

Breakfast:

Cottage cheese with pineapple chunks and a sprinkle of walnuts.

Lunch:

Grilled shrimp tacos in lettucewraps with fresh mango salsa.

Snack:

Hard boiled eggs with a pinch of sea salt

Dinner:

Baked cod with roasted Brussels sprouts and a side of wild rice.

Day 4

Breakfast:

Chia pudding with coconut milk and fresh raspberries.

Lunch:

Mixed greens salad with grilled chicken breast, cherry tomatoes, and olive oildressing.

Snack:

Carrot sticks with guacamole.

Dinner:

Thai basil tofu stir-fry with brown rice

7-Day High Protein, Low Inflammatory, Whole Food Meal Plan (cont.)

Day 5

Breakfast:

Smoothie made with spinach, banana, protein powder, and unsweetenedalmond milk.

Lunch:

Tuna salad on mixed greens with a balsamic vinaigrette.

Snack:

Edamame with a sprinkle of sea salt.

Dinner:

Lemon herb roasted chicken with cauliflower mash and steamed asparagus.

Day 6

Breakfast:

Scrambled eggs with smoked salmon and a side of sliced avocado.

Lunch:

Lentil soup with a side of mixed greens.

Snack:

Apple slices with almond butter.

Dinner:

Baked mackerel with a quinoa and cucumber salad.

Day 7

Breakfast:

Buckwheat pancakes with fresh strawberries and a dollop of Greek yogurt.

Lunch:

Chicken and avocado lettuce wraps with a side of cherry tomatoes.

Snack:

Celery sticks with hummus.

Dinner:

Grilled lamb chops with a roasted vegetable medley and a side of millet.

Ensure each meal and snack is balanced to meet the minimum 100 grams of protein per day. Adjust portion sizes as needed to achieve nutritional goals

Chapter 15

Supplements

In the journey of health, especially during the perimenopausal phase, every day counts. Hormonal imbalance can lead to a vast number of uncomfortable symptoms such as irregular cycles, painful periods, breast pain and mood swings accompanied by cravings. Our last pillar of Aeryon Wellness, we focus on support supplements that can serve as a powerful tool.

Here are the key supplements I have in my daily regime.

MAGNESIUM

Magnesium is an essential mineral the human body cannot produce on its own, making it necessary to obtain through diet or supplementation. Magnesium is vital for perimenopausal women as it supports various bodily functions, including regulating mood, managing anxiety and promoting better sleep quality. It also is key to bone health, working alongside calcium and vitamin D to maintain bone density. It affects more than 300 enzymatic processes, including energy production, nerve function, muscle contractions and maintaining healthy bones.

Despite its importance, modern diets often lack sufficient magnesium due to soil depletion, food processing and lifestyle factors. Magnesium supplementation can help bridge this gap, ensuring the body receives an adequate amount to support optimal health and prevent deficiencies that may lead to issues such as fatigue, muscle cramps and even cardiovascular problems.

Various types of magnesium supplements are available, each with its own characteristics and potential benefits. Here's an overview of different forms of magnesium supplementation and their specific uses:

MAGNESIUM CITRATE	Bound to citric acid, magnesium citrate is well-absorbed but may have a mild laxative effect. It is a suitable choice for general magnesium supplementation and may be helpful for occasional constipation.
MAGNESIUM OXIDE	While magnesium oxide is poorly absorbed in the gastrointestinal tract, it is effective as an antacid and laxative. However, it may not be as efficient in increasing magnesium levels compared to other forms.
MAGNESIUM BISGLYCINATE	Magnesium bisglycinate is well-absorbed and less likely to cause loose stools than citrate and oxide forms. It is suitable for those who don't require a laxative effect but still want optimal magnesium absorption. The glycine component also has calming properties, making it beneficial for promoting sleep.
MAGNESIUM TAURATE	Taurine, an amino acid, helps minimize the laxative effect of magnesium. Magnesium taurate may be advantageous for individuals seeking heart health benefits, as taurine itself has potential cardiovascular benefits. component also has calming properties, making it beneficial for promoting sleep.
MAGNESIUM L-THREONATE	This unique form of magnesium can cross the blood-brain barrier, potentially offering benefits for anxiety, depression and cognition. Its ability to support brain function makes it distinctive among other magnesium forms.

Understanding the different magnesium supplements can help you choose the most appropriate form based on your specific needs and desired outcomes.

IRON

Iron plays a critical role in transporting oxygen throughout the body and supporting energy levels. For perimenopausal women, iron deficiency is an important consideration and common effect as these women may experience changes in menstrual cycles. Adequate iron levels are vital for maintaining cognitive function, as low iron can contribute to fatigue and reduced mental clarity. Additionally, iron supports immune health, helping to protect against illnesses and infections. Incorporating iron-rich foods, such as lean meats, beans and leafy greens, along with supplementing when necessary, can aid in meeting the heightened iron needs during perimenopause.

When it comes to iron supplementation, different types are available, each with its own characteristics and benefits. The most common forms include:

Ferrous Sulfate, which is widely used, readily available and provides a high concentration of elemental iron, making it effective for addressing iron deficiencies.

Iron Bisglycinate is a well-absorbed form of iron that is easily tolerated and less likely to cause digestive discomfort compared to other forms. It is suitable for individuals who are prone to experiencing digestive issues with other types of iron supplements.

Iron Fumarate, also highly absorbable, is commonly used to treat iron deficiency anemia. It provides a higher amount of elemental iron per dose compared to other forms.

Iron supplementation should always be done under the guidance of a healthcare professional, as excessive iron intake can have adverse effects. Your doctor can help determine the appropriate type and dosage of iron supplements based on your individual needs and iron levels.

Recommendations for managing iron deficiency include:

- Know the common signs of iron deficiency. Fatigue, exercise intolerance, cold intolerance, hair loss, dizziness, irritability, brain fog and restless legs are some of the common signs.
- Test ferritin levels regularly. Regular monitoring of ferritin levels can help identify iron deficiency and guide further treatment.
- Discuss low thyroid with your doctor. Low thyroid function can overlap with symptoms of iron deficiency. It's important to discuss both conditions with your doctor, as iron is essential for optimal thyroid function.
- Know your ferritin level. Request your ferritin level from the lab, your doctor or access your test results online. This information will help you have an informed discussion with your pharmacist or healthcare team about your iron supplementation needs.

Remember, proper diagnosis and management of iron deficiency should involve working closely with a healthcare professional to ensure optimal iron levels and overall well-being.

OMEGA-3S

Omega-3 fatty acids, specifically EPA and DHA, offer a range of health benefits for both the heart and the brain. Let's explore the advantages of incorporating omega-3s into your daily routine:

Heart Health

EPA in omega-3s reduces inflammation in our bodies, benefiting not only our joints but also our arteries. Reducing inflammation in the arteries with fish oil — one of the best sources of omega-3s — can significantly decrease the risk of heart attack and stroke, potentially by up to 47%. When inflammation is reduced, the heart can function more efficiently, especially vital for women's health as heart disease is the leading cause of premature death among women.

Brain Function

DHA, another omega-3 fatty acid, plays a crucial role in cognitive function and brain protection. By including omega-3s in your routine, you can prioritize both heart health and brain health. Omega-3s have been shown to enhance cognitive function and may play a role in preventing Alzheimer's disease, as 70% of Alzheimer's patients are women.

Other Benefits

As we age, inflammation can become a more significant factor in our overall well-being, making omega-3s even more essential. These fatty acids can also support joint health, digestive health and overall body wellness.

While it may be challenging to obtain adequate omega-3s from our diet alone, high-quality fish oil supplements can help bridge the gap. Look for supplements that have been thoroughly cleansed to ensure purity and consider vegan options if desired. Consistent intake of omega-3 supplements, usually for six to 12 weeks, is necessary to experience their full benefits.

Incorporating omega-3s into your daily routine can have a transformative impact on your overal wel-being, supporting heart health, brain function and many other aspects of your health. Consult with a natural health advisor to find the best omega-3 supplement for your needs and enjoy the wide-ranging benefits they provide.

VITAMIN D

Vitamin D is critical to maintaining bone health, especially for perimenopausal women who are at an increased risk of osteoporosis due to hormonal changes. It helps to enhance calcium absorption in the gut, which is essential for keeping bones strong and reducing the likelihood of fractures. Beyond bone health, adequate vitamin D levels can improve mood and reduce the risk of depression, which can be particularly beneficial during the emotional fluctuations commonly experienced in perimenopause.

Research also suggests that vitamin D may support cardiovascular health, helping to lower blood pressure and improve overal heart function. Lastly, sufficient vitamin D levels contribute to better immune function, providing additional protection against infections and autoimmune conditions that may become more prevalent during this transition period. Here are some reasons why daily intake of vitamin D is vital:

1
Bone Health

Vitamin D helps regulate calcium and phosphorus levels, promoting optimal bone health and reducing the risk of conditions such as osteoporosis and fractures.

2
Immune Function

Adequate levels of vitamin D support a robust immune system, helping the body defend against infections, viruses and diseases.

3
Mood and Mental Health

Research suggests a link between vitamin D deficiency and mood disorders such as depression and seasonal affective disorder (SAD). Sustaining sufficient levels of vitamin D may contribute to improved mood and mental wel-being.

4
Heart Health

Vitamin D is believed to play a role in maintaining cardiovascular health, including helping to regulate blood pressure and reducing the risk of heart diseases.

5
Cancer Prevention

Some studies suggest that vitamin D may have a protective effect against certain types of cancer, including colorectal, breast and prostate cancers.

Given the inadequate sun exposure in many regions and the challenge of obtaining sufficient vitamin D from dietary sources alone, daily supplementation becomes crucial. Supplementing with G'Day Sunshine Vitamin D 2500 can ensure you are getting the RDA of vitamin D. Consult with a healthcare professional to determine the right dosage and form of vitamin D supplementation for your specific needs. By ensuring optimal vitamin D levels, you can support your overal health and wel-being.

PROTEIN POWDERS

Whey and vegan protein powders offer a convenient way to meet daily protein needs, which is essential for muscle repair and growth. Whey protein is quickly absorbed by the body, making it an excellent option for post-workout recovery, while vegan protein sources provide a plant based alternative that is often easier to digest for the lactose intolerance.

Additionally, vegan protein powders typically contain a broader range of nutrients, including fibre and antioxidants, which support overal health. Incorporating either type of protein powder can help with weight management by promoting satiety and reducing hunger. Ultimately, the choice between whey and vegan protein may come down to dietary preferences and individual health goals.

CREATINE

Creatine is a naturally occurring compound that is primarily found in red meat and fish. It is synthesized in the body from three amino acids: arginine, glycine and methionine, predominantly in the liver, kidneys and pancreas. The synthesis process involves a series of enzymatic reactions that convert these amino acids into phosphocreatine, which is stored in the muscles and plays a critical role in the production of adenosine triphosphate (ATP)—the energy currency of the cell. Approximately 95% of the body's creatine is stored in skeletal muscle, while the remaining 5% is found in the brain, heart and other tissues. For those who may have dietary restrictions or do not consume enough creatine through their diet, supplementation with B Strong Creatine for Women can provide a convenient way to increase their creatine levels.

You lose muscle mass starting at the age of 30 at a rate of three to five percent per decade, with the decline accelerating after the age of 60. Incorporating five grams of creatine monohydrate daily, along with added resistance training, has been proven to counteract some of this muscle loss. Research shows that this combination not only helps preserve lean muscle mass but also enhances strength and performance in older adults. By supporting muscle regeneration and energy production, creatine supplementation can help your body maintain mobility and overall physical health in aging populations.

Additionally, creatine may assist in managing Type 2 diabetes, a condition that affects how the body utilizes insulin, particularly in middle-aged and older individuals. Emerging studies also suggest that creatine may benefit individuals with certain neurological diseases, such as Parkinson's and Alzheimer's, though its effectiveness during advanced stages of these disorders remains uncertain. For women in and beyond the menopause transition, research finds that creatine supplementation can help counteract the menopause-related decline in muscle, bone and strength by reducing inflammation, oxidative stress, and serum markers of bone resorption, while also resulting in an increase in bone formation.

When incorporating creatine supplementation and resistance training into a fitness regimen, some individuals may experience an increase in the number on the scale. However, this weight gain is often due to water and development of muscle tissue, as muscle weighs more than fat.

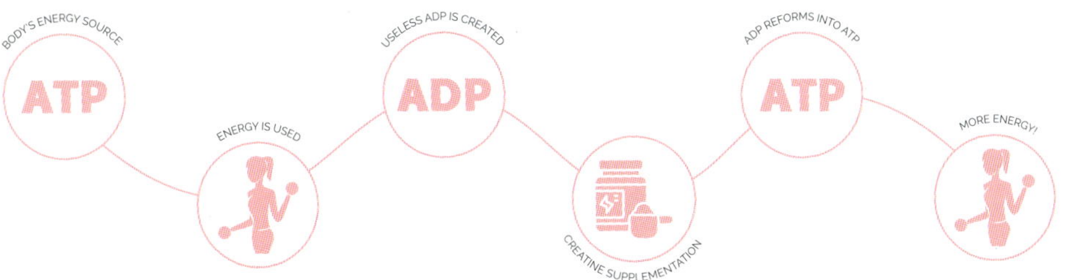
BODY'S ENERGY SOURCE
ATP
ENERGY IS USED
USELESS ADP IS CREATED
ADP
CREATINE SUPPLEMENTATION
ADP REFORMS INTO ATP
ATP
MORE ENERGY!

As muscle mass increases, it can lead to a healthier, leaner body composition, improving overall strength and metabolic function. Unlike fat gain, which can contribute to health issues, the increase in muscle mass is beneficial as it supports physical performance and enhances the body's ability to burn calories at rest. Therefore, while the scale might show a higher number, the underlying changes in body composition are often positive and reflect improved health outcomes. This is where using waist-to-hip circumference measurements can be best used to determine results.

Chapter 16

Sleep

Sleep is a foundational pillar of health, and its significance during perimenopause and beyond cannot be overstated. This transitional time of life brings hormonal shifts, such as fluctuating estrogen and progesterone levels, that can directly affect sleep quality. Many women experience challenges like insomnia, night sweats or waking up frequently during the night, leaving them feeling exhausted and unrefreshed. These issues can be compounded by the demands of career, family and other responsibilities, making consistent rest feel elusive.

Prioritizing sleep is one of the most empowering steps you can take for your well being during midlife. Simple but impactful habits, such as maintaining a regular sleep schedule, creating a calming bedtime routine and limiting screen time before bed, can help improve sleep quality. For those facing persistent difficulties, consulting with a healthcare provider can provide additional solutions, including addressing underlying conditions or considering tailored treatments.

Quality sleep is not just about physical rejuvenation. It's also a key factor in emotional resilience, mental clarity and overall vitality. By committing to rest and recovery, you're giving yourself the tools to thrive in this vibrant phase of life

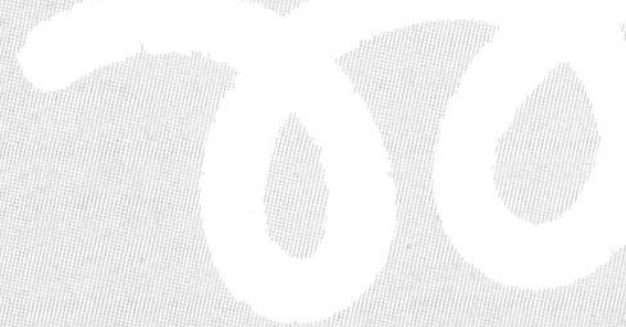

PERIMENOPAUSE AND SLEEP

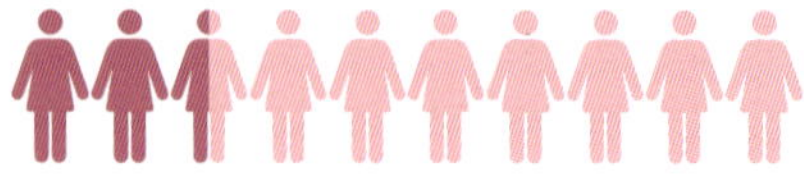

1 in 4 perimenopausal women have trouble falling asleep.

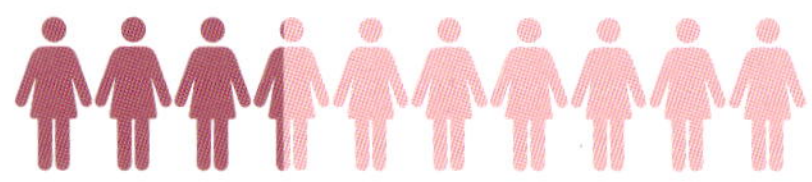

1 in 3 women have trouble staying asleep, waking up multiple times per night.

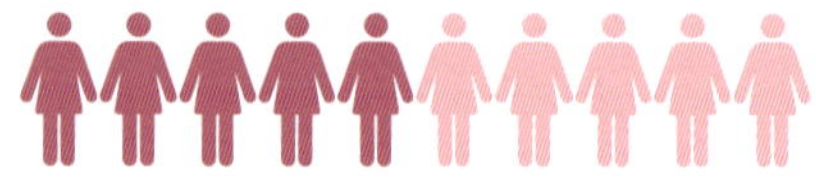

Half of all perimenopausal women sleep less than 7 hours per night.

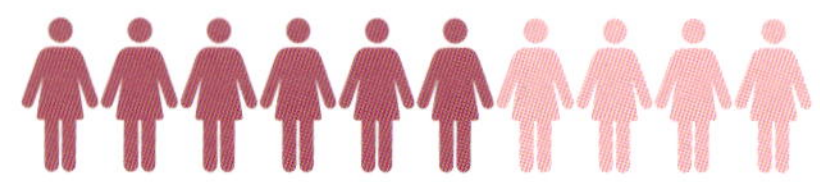

Over half wake up feeling tired more than 4 days a week.

FIVE KEY PRACTICES FOR A GOOD NIGHT'S SLEEP

1

Establish a Regular Sleep Schedule:

Going to bed and waking up at the same time every day, even on weekends, helps regulate your body's internal clock, making it easier to fall asleep and stay asleep.

3

Optimize Your Sleep Environment:

Ensure your bedroom is cool, dark and quiet. Investing in a comfortable mattress and pillows can also dramatically improve the quality of your sleep.

2

Create a Relaxing Bedtime Routine:

Engaging in calming activities such as reading, meditating or taking a warm bath before bed can signal to your brain that it's time to wind down

4
Be Mindful of Diet and Caffeine:

Avoid heavy meals, alcohol and caffeine close to bedtime. These can interfere with sleep by disrupting your circadian rhythm or causing discomfort.

5
Limit Screen Time Before Bed:

The blue light emitted by phones, tablets and computers affects melatonin production, making it harder to fall asleep. Aim to disconnect from screens at least an hour before bed.

Progesterone, often referred to as a "calming hormone," plays a significant role in promoting restful sleep, especially for women in midlife. This hormone has natural sedative effects, helping to relax the body and mind, which can ease the process of falling and staying asleep. During perimenopause and menopause, progesterone levels may decline, contributing to sleep disruptions. Supplementing with progesterone, under the guidance of a healthcare professional, can often restore balance and improve sleep quality.

Additionally, natural supplements can further support better sleep. Melatonin, known for regulating the sleep-wake cycle, is a common choice for easing sleep onset. Magnesium, particularly in the form of magnesium glycinate, has calming effects on the nervous system and supports muscle relaxation. Snooze is a melatonin-free, all natural, non-addictive sleep support supplement has well known soothing properties to ensure a restful night's sleep.

By prioritizing these habits and recognizing the importance of restorative sleep, you can greatly improve your overall health and quality of life during midlife and beyond.

Chapter 17

WHI Disservice

The Women's Health Initiative (WHI) study conducted in 2002 cast a shadow of doubt over hormone therapy, leading to widespread fear and misconception about its potential risks. However, the study itself had several flaws and failed to communicate all the benefits of hormone therapy effectively. The study focused on non-bioidentical hormone therapy, studying women between the ages of 50 and 71, a demographic more susceptible to heart disease and breast cancer due to age alone. The early results, including the increased risk of blood clots, heart disease, stroke and breast cancer, were expected but were not presented in the context of age-related risks. The negative headlines resulted in many physicians discontinuing hormone therapy for their patients, despite the flaws in the study.

In 2017, the North American Menopause Society (NAMS) released updated guidelines stating that hormone therapy is safe when an individualized risk assessment is conducted. The guidelines recommend starting hormone therapy within 10 years of menopause and before the age of 60. However, there is no universal guideline for the duration of hormone therapy, and decisions should be made on an individual basis with the guidance of a healthcare professional.

Be aware of the misinformation surrounding hormone therapy and consult reliable sources and healthcare professionals for accurate information when making decisions about your hormone health.

Whether you choose natural supplementation, menopause hormone therapy (MHT) or another approach that works for you, the goal is to align with what makes you feel your best. However, it is equally important to reflect on the daily habits that influence your overal wellbeing. Nutrition, physical activity, stress management, and quality sleep are key pillars that shape your health and vitality. By cultivating positive daily practices, you create a foundation for the best version of yourself, a lowing any chosen interventions or therapies to work more effectively in supporting your goals.

Chapter 18

Menopause Hormone Therapy

Menopausal hormone therapy (MHT), also known as hormone replacement therapy (HRT), offers a range of benefits for individuals experiencing menopause-related symptoms. MHT can help alleviate hot flashes, night sweats, mood swings and other discomforts by supplementing hormone levels that naturally decline during this stage of life. MHT is designed to support women's health during midlife and is prescribed after conducting an individualized risk assessment. The key considerations when prescribing hormone therapy are the appropriate hormones, optimal dosage and suitable mode of delivery for each individual.

The most prescribed hormones in MHT are progesterone and estrogen. Testosterone and DHEA may also be a part of an individual hormone therapy protocol. The timing of hormone therapy depends on factor such as age and stage (in terms of time since the last period) and it is important to note that women in perimenopause may require just progesterone to support symptoms. Have a conversation with your Practioner about the benefits of progesterone, regardless of whether a woman has a uterus as progesterone place multiple roles beyond protecting the uterine lining.

It is also important to clarify common terms that can lead to confusion when discussing hormone therapy, such as bioidentical versus non-bioidentical, synthetic, natural, compounded, FDA-approved/Health Canada approved and progestins versus progesterone.

BIOIDENTICAL VERSUS NON-BIOIDENTICAL HORMONES

Bioidentical hormones, also referred to as "body-identical," are manufactured in laboratories but have a molecular structure identical to the hormones naturally produced by the human body. This similarity allows bioidentical hormones to function in a way that closely mimics the body's own hormones. Commercially available bioidentical hormones have been approved by regulatory bodies like the FDA or Health Canada, ensuring specific standards of quality and safety. On the other hand, compounded bioidentical hormones, which are created by specialized pharmacies to meet individual patient needs, are not regulated or approved by these agencies, which may raise concerns around their consistency and safety.

SYNTHETIC VERSUS NATURAL HORMONES

The terms "synthetic" and "natural" are often misunderstood in the context of hormone therapy. Historically, "synthetic" referred to non-bioidentical hormones, such as those used in older studies like the WHI, which included hormones made from ingredients dissimilar to the ones naturally produced by the human body. However, the truth is that all hormone therapy products—whether bioidentical or not—are manufactured in a laboratory and thus technically synthetic. The term "natural" more accurately refers to the hormones that a woman's body produces on its own. Ultimately, distinguishing hormones by bioidentical versus non bioidentical provides a clearer and more accurate understanding.

COMPOUNDING

Compounding refers to the process of customizing medications to suit the unique needs of a patient. This is often carried out by compounding pharmacies, where pharmacists adjust or reformulate medications to create specific dosages or formats that are not commercially available. For instance, a medication available only in 100 milligram capsules might be compounded into a liquid, gummy or a custom dose, such as 150 milligrams, to better match a patient's requirements.

Compounding is commonly seen in situations involving special dosing needs or alternative administration methods, like for children or pets. However, compounded therapies are not FDA or Health Canada-approved because their unique, personalized nature makes them difficult to standardize and regulate. While compounding offers valuable versatility, it is vital for patients to consult closely with their healthcare provider to ensure safety and efficacy.

Understanding these distinctions is critical for making informed decisions about hormone therapy, as each approach carries its unique benefits and considerations depending on individual health needs.

Mode of delivery refers to the method by which hormone therapy is administered, such as orally, trans dermally through the skin or vaginally. The prescribing physician typically determines the most appropriate method based on health research, considering which mode offers the most effective outcomes or the safest profile for the patient. Additionally, the mode of delivery may be selected after discussing patient preferences, responses or compliance with the therapy to ensure optimal treatment results.

Many of us hope for a "magic pill" or a "one-size-fits-all" solution, which is completely understandable. However, when it comes to health—especially women's health and hormone health—the process is rarely that simple. With hormone therapy, it's essential to schedule regular review appointments with your prescribing physician. These appointments allow you to discuss your experiences, both positive and any potential negative effects. Adjustments and fine-tuning are often necessary to ensure the therapy is tailored to your specific needs. After all, the goal of hormone therapy is for you to feel your very best!

Ultimately, a review appointment with the prescribing physician is crucial to discuss experiences and make any necessary adjustments or tweaks to the hormone therapy protocol, as the goal is for individuals to feel amazing with hormone therapy.

When it comes to health—especially women's health and hormone health—the process is rarely a one-size-fits-all solution.

Chapter 19

Final Thoughts

Navigating perimenopause is a deeply personal and evolving experience, unique to each individual. While it brings challenges such as hormonal shifts, sleep disruptions and physical changes, it also provides an opportunity to prioritize self-care and rediscover personal strength. By understanding the biological processes at play and proactively seeking tailored solutions, you can confidently face this transitional phase.

Remember, perimenopause is not an end but rather a beginning—a chance to forge a healthier, more balanced lifestyle and to cultivate greater awareness of your body's needs. With the right tools, support and mindset, this period can be a time of empowerment and renewal.

Working with a practitioner who specializes in hormonal health can be an invaluable step during perimenopause. These professionals can provide tailored guidance and personalized treatment options that align with your unique needs and goals. Whether it's through testing to better understand your hormonal changes, recommending therapies to address specific symptoms, or offering nutritional and lifestyle advice, a skilled practitioner can help you navigate this transition with greater confidence and clarity.

Partnering with someone knowledgeable ensures that you are supported every step of the way, empowering you to make informed choices about your health and well-being.

It is my hope that this guide has provided you with meaningful insights, practical strategies and a sense of encouragement as you take this next step in your life's journey. Remember, you are not alone — millions of individuals share this path, and together, we can create a supportive and informed community that makes perimenopause less daunting and more empowering.

Chapter 20

Aeryon Wellness Supplements & Glossary

As we have spoken in this book, navigating perimenopause is a deeply personal and often complex journey, one that challenges us to listen to our bodies and prioritize our well-being. Through the ups and downs, remember that you are not alone, and resources, tools and communities are available every step of the way to support you.

Aeryon Wellness exists because of this shared experience—because women deserve access to effective, trustworthy supplements crafted with their unique needs in mind. While there is no magic pill, there is power in knowledge, self-care, and using products that align with your health goals.

I am immensely proud of what we have built—an award-winning line of products that not only meet the highest standards but are designed with care, compassion and a commitment to empowering women. This section contains a glossary of our products, each paired with a QR code that links to our wellness program, accessible directly on every product label. Additionally, you'll find videos explaining the distinctive benefits and properties of each supplement, helping you make informed choices for your health and well-being.

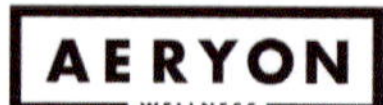

EMPOWERING WOMEN WITH HOLISTIC HEALTH

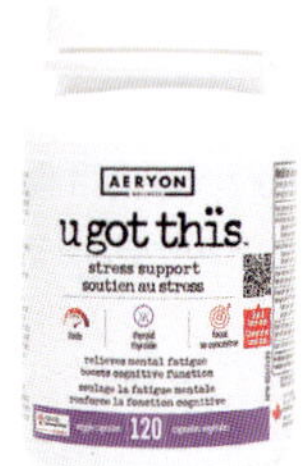

U GOT THÏS

- Reduces Mental Stress (Rhodiola)
- Supports Libido & Cognition (Panex Ginseng)
- Supports Liver & Energy (Schisandra)
- Reduces Cortisol & Stress Support (KSM66 Ashwagandha)
- Immune Supportive (Reishi Mushroom)

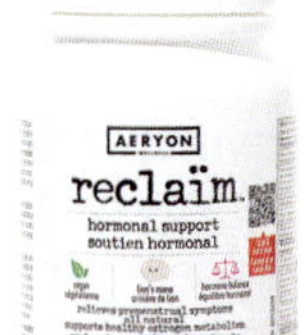

RECLAÏM

- Prevents Breast, Prostate and Colon Cancer (DIM)
- Mood and Memory (Lions Mane)
- Supports Ovulation and Production of Luteinizing Hormone (Chastetree)
- Supports Estrogen Metabolism (Broccoli Sulforaphane)
- Immune Support (Astralagus and Zinc)

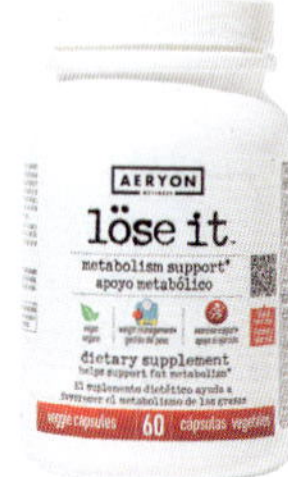

LÖSE IT

- Promotes Estrogen Balance (Indol 3 - Carbinol)
- Low Stimulant (Less than 1 cup of coffee per serving)
- Increases Metabolism (Red Pepper Extract)
- Supports Muscle Recovery (L-Carnitine)
- Suppresses Appetite (Olive Leaf)
- Excellent Pre-Workout/Energy Support

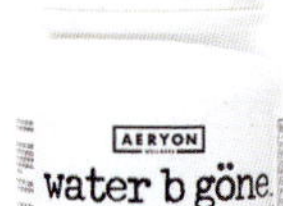

WATER B GÖNE

- Relieves Bloating
- Salty Meal Solution
- Reduces Water Retention
- Diuretic Support (Clinical dose Dandelion 4:1 Extract)
- UTI Solution (Clinical dose of Juniper Berry 4: 1 Extract)
- Supports PMS, Menopausal Symptoms (Black Cohosh)
- Prevents Cramping (Magnesium)

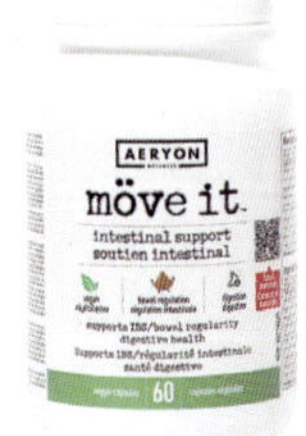

MÖVE IT

- Constipation/Healthy Bowel Support
- Non Habit Forming
- Inflammation Support (Boswellia)
- Promote Growth of Good Bacteria (Cape Aloe)
- Stool Softener (Magnesium Hydroxide)
- Restore the Integrity of the Gut (Marshmallow)

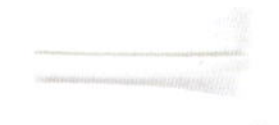

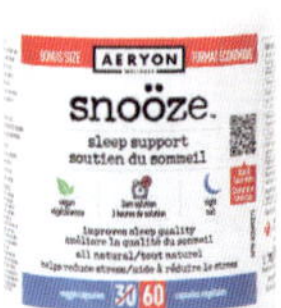

SNOÖZE

- Melatonin Free
- No Sleepy Hangover
- Reduces Stress & Anxiety (L-Theanine)
- Heart Health (Hawthorn)
- Helps with Nights Sweats (Passionflower)
- Relaxes and Reduces GABA Breakdown (Valerian)

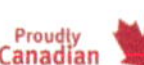

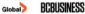

RESOURCES

To create "Navigating Perimenopause" with accuracy and relevance, we referenced a variety of reputable resources. Key sources included peer-reviewed medical journals, studies from institutions specializing in women's health, and expert recommendations from gynecologists and endocrinologists. Additionally, we incorporated insights from books written by healthcare professionals and organizations such as the North American Menopause Society (NAMS). These materials provided a comprehensive foundation for understanding the physiological, emotional and lifestyle changes associated with perimenopause.

- Lisa Mosconi, PHD The Menopause Brain
- Dr. Mary Claire Haver, The New Menopause
- Dr Jen Gunter, The Menopause Manifesto
- Dr Vonda Wright, Fitness After 40
- Dr Gabrielle Lyon, Forever Strong
- https://menopausefoundationcanada.ca
- https://www.hopkinsmedicine.org/health/conditions-and-diseases/
- perimenopause
- https://menopause.org
- https://www.healthlinkbc.ca/healthwise/menopause-and-
- perimenopause
- https://www.health.harvard.edu/womens-health/perimenopause-rocky-
- road-to-menopause
- https://my.clevelandclinic.org/health/diseases/21608-perimenopause
- https://www.ncbi.nlm.nih.gov/pmc/articles/PMC10273865/
- https://www.mayoclinic.org/diseases-conditions/menopause/ diagnosis-treatment/drc 20353401#:~:text=You%20can%20get%20home%20tests,fall%20during%20 your%20menstrual%20cycle

NOTES

NOTES

NOTES